Bipolar not ADHD

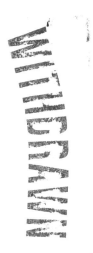

Bipolar not ADHD

Unrecognized epidemic of manic depressive illness in children

George Isaac, MD

Writers Club Press
San Jose New York Lincoln Shanghai

Contents

INTRODUCTION

Manic-depressive illness, otherwise known as bipolar disorder, is the single, most troublesome, and most prevalent psychiatric illness of children brought to our psychiatric clinics today for emotional and behavioral problems. This opinion is primarily based on my observations and clinical studies, which I undertook during the past three decades. Few people are aware that this illness is widely prevalent among our children, and is arguably, the main reason for severe, persistent emotional turmoil, aggression, and out of control behavior in children and adolescents

This book is an attempt to make people become more aware, of the extremely, frequent occurrence of bipolar disorder in children and the fact that it is seldom recognized for what it is. My hope is that better recognition of this devastating illness will lead to better care of the children who suffer from it, intensive research efforts, and better remedies.

If the high prevalence of this illness in children and the turmoil it creates continue to go unrecognized, it could even result in serious disintegration of our society. Such a situation may occur because children affected by this illness not only suffer intense emotional agony, but their dysfunctional state and behavioral problems–often out of control and unmanageable–produce a disastrous ripple effect on their family and others involved with them in school and elsewhere. Also, most such children become dysfunctional adults, unable to support themselves, sustain lasting relationships, and prone to a life of substance abuse and involvement in crimes. A great deal of social turmoil is the inevitable result.

The high prevalence of bipolar disorder among our troubled children and the lack of awareness of it among mental health and other professionals who deal with such children are shocking indeed. The inability of child psychiatrists, psychiatrists, other mental health professionals, and pediatricians–the professionals who are primarily responsible for the treatment of such children–to recognize the manifestations of this illness, in my experience, is nothing short of shocking.

Most clinicians misunderstand the manifestations of bipolar disorder in children for attention deficit hyperactivity disorder (ADHD), or conduct disorder, or other related problems [1,22, 23. 24]. They do so because it has been,—and still is-, the erroneous manner in which such children and their problems were misunderstood in psychiatry–especially in American Psychiatry. Often children who suffer from bipolar disorder are misunderstood to be exhibiting bad behavior due to faulty upbringing, or just reacting to—or rebelling against—unhappy occurrences or circumstances in their life. The fact that they suffer from a serious illness caused by abnormalities of their brain chemistry, seldom occur, to professionals and others who deal with them.

This book is an attempt to make psychiatric, medical, and other professionals who deal with children, and society as a whole, become aware of how common and serious a problem bipolar disorder in children is. Better awareness and identification are essential before intensive research efforts to understand the genetic and biochemical etiology of this illness could occur, as a high priority. Such efforts are essential, as the treatments available today for this illness–especially in children–are extremely inadequate, and only through research efforts could effective, if not curative, treatments could be developed. To make people aware of how common this illness is among our troubled children and youth—yet how unrecognized and misdiagnosed it is—and help our health professionals identify and diagnose this disorder in a highly competent manner, are the main objectives of this book.

In this book, the terms "bipolar disorder," and "manic-depressive illness," are used interchangeably (as they denote the same illness—bipolar disorder being the modern term). However, neither of these terms, I believe, aptly describes the nature of the illness or its symptomatology because of its varied and complex manifestations.

This book is mainly based on knowledge and insights I gained during the past three decades as a, child and adult psychiatrist involved in the evaluation and treatment of severely, emotionally and behaviorally troubled children and adults. A good majority of the children and adults I have evaluated and treated during these decades, suffered from recognized and unrecognized forms of bipolar disorder. It is the plight of children who suffer from the forms of bipolar disorder, which have gone unrecognized that prompted me to write this book.

I have made an attempt to explain why I consider this illness to be extremely prevalent in children, and also, why it has gone unrecognized and mistaken for problems such as ADHD, conduct disorder, oppositional defiant disorder [2], and other problems. Since this illness is most often mistaken for ADHD and conduct disorder, issues regarding such misdiagnosis, and how to minimize such mistakes are dealt with, whenever appropriate. Such discussions and clarifications which occur repeatedly throughout the book is intended to help the reader become intensely aware of the tendency for misdiagnosis and competent in accurately identifying this illness in children.

The common manifestations of the illness—its signs and symptoms—as they occur in children are listed and discussed, as well as practical suggestions given to help identify the illness in children. Though not the primary objective of this book, a brief discussion of the possible etiology of this illness, and a chapter giving practical suggestions regarding treatment are also included (though I consider treatment available for this illness today—especially for children-, woefully inadequate).

The widespread occurrence of this illness in children and the past, and continuing tendency to misdiagnose it as ADHD, conduct disorder, and the like, calls into question, most of the research that has been conducted on ADHD and related disorders until now. I came to this conclusion because of the fact that a high number of children with bipolar disorder would have been misdiagnosed as suffering from ADHD, conduct disorder, and the like, and included among such research subjects erroneously, and hence, the findings arrived upon in many such studies may not be valid.

This book is not a comprehensive treatise on manic-depressive or bipolar disorder in children. Hence, theoretical discussions are kept to a minimum. It is clear at present that, this illness is primarily a genetic illness caused by abnormal gene or genes and the resulting biochemical problems that adversely affect brain function. Only brief mention is made of this topic of the etiology of the illness, as it is not the primary purpose of this book, and also because, very little is known that is definite about the genetic and biochemical factors that cause this illness. [34]

In this book, the term 'child' is used, in general, to refer to both younger (pre-pubertal) children and adolescents. When there is a special need to refer to younger children or adolescents separately, it is done so in a manner that makes it clear as to which particular age group is being specifically referred to.

In my opinion, this illness is so prevalent among our troubled youngsters, and yet, so misunderstood, that such lack of recognition itself is one of the major causes of disruption and chaos in our schools and communities today. Few of the children who suffer from this illness or their parents receive the understanding and support they deserve, because, professionals—including those in mental health, medicine, education, the legal system, and other relevant fields, have little awareness of the high prevalence or manifestations of this illness among children they deal with. The plight of these children and their parents are seldom understood. I have come to recognize that, a great deal of social turmoil and misery are directly and indirectly caused by this illness and the fact that it is seldom understood for what it is. Many of the children are misunderstood and mistreated; many end up in jails, or become homeless as they reach adulthood, if not earlier. Many grow up to be highly dysfunctional adults. Many go through their whole life misunderstood as bad people or as people who do not want to help themselves, receiving little assistance or understanding they deserve.

Today, with the all-out attempts to shrink the welfare roll, and the attempt by Social Security Administration to make it more difficult to obtain disability benefits, many such people have no place to turn to for assistance they truly deserve. As a result, many young people who suffer from this illness are more prone to turn to a life of crime. This illness and the dysfunction it causes, make most adults who suffer from it unable to work consistently and earn a living. Once the extent and seriousness of this illness in the population is truly recognized, our criteria to provide social assistance, social security disability benefits, and other assistances will have to be significantly modified to include this population of children and adults suffering from unrecognized bipolar disorder. A great deal of commitment and resources will be needed to accomplish this. The reality of pervasive disability among this large population that suffers from unrecognized bipolar disorder cannot be ignored for too long in a civilized society such as ours. Today, when, even experienced psychiatrists fail to recognize this illness in many, it is no wonder that such agencies reject the requests for assistance of many who are suffering from this illness, assuming they are fit to work and earn a living. Perhaps, awareness brought on by publications such as this will help, at least to some degree, to rectify the misunderstandings about this illness–especially in children—which are prevalent among those who occupy important decision making positions.

I present this book, as part of an attempt to make people become more aware of the magnitude of the problem of bipolar disorder in children, so that, as a community we will rise-up to address the challenge posed by this illness. Mainly, I hope for better identification of the illness, better treatment, support for the parents and families, and most importantly—intensified research to develop a cure for this illness. In my opinion, this illness deserves at least the attention and urgency, illnesses such as cancer and heart disease receive. Given the suffering and social catastrophe this illness causes, only the problem of AIDS seems to deserve a higher priority today.

The interest in writing this book originated with a few clinical studies I did more than a decade ago, when I first started becoming aware of the widespread occurrence of unrecognized bipolar disorder in children.[22,23,24] At that time, few child psychiatrists—let alone others—recognized the high prevalence and manifestations of this illness in children. My three papers on this subject based on that work and published several years ago [2,23,24] forms the background for this book and are reprinted in the appendix for ease of reference, as they are frequently cited in this book and may be worthwhile reading for more than one reason.

I note with some satisfaction, how, many publishers and psychiatric experts, a decade back, did not want to believe that my observations that this illness was much more prevalent–even extremely common—in children than most people had recognized until then, had merit. The widespread belief among psychiatrists and others then was, that this illness was very rare in children.[7,17] Now, more than ten years later, I note with some satisfaction that the situation is beginning to change—albeit very slowly. Today, at least some leaders in the field have started acknowledging the high prevalence of this illness in children. Advertisements for seminars to educate the professionals about this illness in children are increasingly visible in journals (though such efforts still reveal that even many leaders in the field are quite unclear about the nature of the problem).

I am indebted to all the children who suffer from this illness and their families I was privileged to come to know during the past three decades, from whom I gained invaluable insights about this illness and its impact on them. It is their unrecognized suffering and misunderstood problems that motivated me to write this brief presentation, so that a better future for them and all who suffer from the various forms of this illness may come about. There is little doubt in my mind that most children who suffer from this illness today are misunderstood, and as a result, more often than not, they grow up into a life of turmoil. Many become homeless; many commit suicide; many live a life involved in serious crimes and are imprisoned time and again. Many, even end up in our expanding death rows. Only greater awareness of this illness—especially as it occurs in children-, will help rectify such tragic situation.

I have made all attempts to shield the identity of patients, whose brief case histories or statements are used occasionally in the text to illustrate one point or another. Points or ideas that I consider to be very important are highlighted in bold letters within the text, when appropriate.

CHAPTER I

THE UNRECOGNIZED EPIDEMIC

A catastrophic epidemic of manic-depressive illness or bipolar disorder has been occurring in the children of United States. Yet, few of us are aware of it, and even fewer, the magnitude of the problem.

Children who suffer from this illness are often misunderstood and mistreated because of our lack of awareness. Our schools are seriously affected by the impact of this illness. A large proportion, if not the majority of children, in the special education programs for emotionally and behaviorally disturbed children are affected by this illness and are there because of the effects of this illness. Our family courts and juvenile justice systems are over-run by the effects of this illness on the children they deal with. A large number of children who suffer from this illness come to our child psychiatric clinics and psychiatric in-patient units. Yet, the majority of caregivers in these settings have very little awareness of the nature or seriousness of these children's illness. Our psychiatrists, pediatricians, psychologists, and social workers are dealing with vast numbers of such children every day, but seldom are they aware what ails these children. They are often misdiagnosed, and the misguided treatment provided because of such misdiagnosis, is mostly ineffective—at times even harmful—to these children. We look for reasons for their troubles and troubled behavior, solely, in the inadequacies of their parents or in their socio-economic environment, and totally fail to consider the crucial issue. The crucial issue is the fact that, by and large, what appears to be described vaguely as behavioral and emotional problems of these children—the problems that won't just go away in spite of our run-of-the-mill, though well meaning interventions—are actually manifestations of a sinister mental illness, one that is rooted in the genetics and biology of these suffering children! Our attempts to explain the problems and sufferings of these children, as due to poor parenting, or socioeconomic problems, misses the crucial point that they are actually suffering from bipolar disorder or illness and in effect, worsen the life and problems of these children. I do not mean to imply, however, that an identification of the illness for what it truly is, will just transform their lives to one of tranquil existence, but that not recognizing the problem for what it is, perpetuates or worsens the situation by subjecting them to measures and remedies that are of little benefit or may even be dangerous.

In the following pages I make an attempt to illustrate the point that we have a national catastrophe at hand, that needs recognition by all concerned, if we are to help these children and their families and prevent society itself from disintegrating further by the havoc caused by this illness.

As mentioned in the introduction, this publication is a small attempt to help people, including professionals who deal with children, become more aware of the nature of bipolar disorder in children. Specifically, it is intended for medical and mental health professionals to develop the skills necessary to correctly identify this illness when it occurs in children and deal with the children who suffer from this illness, and their families, in a sensitive, supportive, and effective manner. A cadre of professionals, who are fully aware of the manifestations of this illness in children and truly concerned about its impact on them, is necessary to bring about improvement in the plight of these children. Such awareness and concern by large groups of people are needed, for society—especially those in higher decision-making positions—to become cognizant of the gravity and urgency of the situation. Such awareness is necessary, so that, not only the children who suffer from this illness are understood and treated in the manner they deserve, but also to have adequate resources channeled into research efforts to develop better treatment and preventive measures. Unless health professionals, public at large, and those in charge of allocating funds for medical research and services become aware of the magnitude of the problem of this illness in children, the sorry state of affairs we have today will continue or even worsen. With the strong possibility of the number of people affected by this illness—yet misunderstood and mistreated–increasing, generation after generation, there is even the real danger of a serious disintegration of our society.

Until very recently, the majority of people involved in the care of children with behavioral and emotional problems, failed to recognize that bipolar disorder is very common among such children. The conventional wisdom was that it is extremely rare for children to suffer from this disorder.[7,17] Even in the mid 1990s, publications from prestigious centers continued to make statements that bipolar disorder was "rare but possible in children and adolescents,"[7] revealing the prevailing belief that the illness is a rarity in children. During the past five years or so, there has been a bit more acknowledgement—at least from a few more leaders in the field-, that this illness (which is one of the major mental illnesses) occurs more frequently in children than what was and is still believed to be true. But still, most people involved in the care of severely troubled children, fail to recognize this illness, as they continue to have little awareness that it occurs very frequently in children who are troubled by or manifest significant emotional and behavioral problems. Psychiatric evaluation and treatment reports, from even major academic centers, more often than not, reveal, that their psychiatrists and other clinicians have little awareness that many of the children they are dealing with are actually suffering from this disorder and that, it is the reason for such children's behavioral and emotional problems. It is the rule rather than the exception today that, most children who suffer from this disorder are improperly diagnosed, misunderstood, and receive improper treatment as a result, even though they have been in treatment with various professionals, hospitals, and clinics, often for years. This is true of all school age children—both prepubertal and adolescent.[22,23,24]

An Illness Comes to Focus Slowly

During the late 1960s and early 1970s when I was undergoing training to become a psychiatrist and child psychiatrist, I came to recognize that most children who were brought to the child psychiatric clinics and in-patient units for severe behavioral problems, such as excessive aggression, defiance of adult authority, and persistent out of control behavior, etc., in general, failed to improve significantly in spite of years of treatment efforts. This appeared to be true in our psychiatric centers in general–even the most reputable ones-, where these children often spend years, only to come out as troubled and dysfunctional adults. Most of these children received a diagnosis of hyperkinetic syndrome (known today as attention deficit hyperactivity disorder or ADHD), or conduct disorder. They often received Ritalin (methylphenidate), along with psychotherapeutic efforts, including group therapy and behavior modification measures. Their treatment was difficult because the very nature of their problems made them uncooperative, and the treatment methods available did not seem to be effective in most cases. Many of these children spent years in inpatient units and residential treatment settings (there was no "managed care" then, to limit how many days they could stay in such facilities), but few seemed to benefit from these efforts. During those years, any child experiencing or exhibiting hallucinations or delusions almost automatically got a diagnosis of schizophrenia—a situation that has also not changed much since then. Even in major psychiatric centers, one hardly saw a pre-pubertal child diagnosed as having manic-depressive illness (today's bipolar disorder), during those days. Even among adolescents it was a very rare diagnosis. The diagnosis of this disorder in children was so rare that, many doctors training to become child psychiatrists went through their whole training period without ever having diagnosed, or treated a child with this illness.

Most psychiatrists and child psychiatrists believed that manic-depressive illness was an extremely rare condition in young children, well into the 1990s,[7, 17] and even today. Only if a child exhibited classical signs of mania, such as extreme elation or euphoria, fantastic or grandiose beliefs that appeared to be a sure sign of mental illness to even lay people, flight of ideas, over-activity to the point of not being able to rest or sleep, was manic-depressive illness considered the diagnosis in children during those years. Children who were diagnosed as manic-depressive during those years, had to appear so ill and bizarre in their behavior and utterances that, even people with little knowledge or training in psychiatry would have had little difficulty recognizing them to be acutely and severely mentally ill. Now, at least some of us know from years of experience and observation, that **many manic-depressive children, often, do not exhibit such classical features of the illness, but are nevertheless seriously affected by it in one form or another.**

Looking back at those times, I clearly remember many children who were considered to suffer from hyperkinetic disorder (ADHD) or conduct disorder, year after year, by the psychiatrists who treated them, but who, in retrospect, actually were suffering from bipolar or manic-depressive illness, albeit, at times in its atypical forms (described in detail later). Even though, signs indicating that they actually suffered from this illness would have been evident on careful scrutiny, few of these children were understood to be suffering from this illness at that time. The reasons for such mistakes and failure to recognize the illness are many.

Since child psychiatry was a very new field three decades back, there was only a very limited knowledge base and very limited follow up data available on children who came to treatment. There was little awareness of the myriad manifestations of manic-depressive illness in adults–and even less so in children. Because of these and related other reasons, even experienced clinicians did not suspect or recognize this disorder in children when it continued to unfold in front of them, time and again.

As I went through the 1970s and '80s as a psychiatrist and child psychiatrist here in the U.S., Canada, and India, it dawned on me—as well as some others-[2, 8, 9, 10, 26, 29,39,40] that not only was bipolar disorder misdiagnosed as schizophrenia in adults, that such misdiagnosis was extremely common in adolescents and children as well. I also started becoming more and more aware that manic-depressive illness may be quite common in adolescents and even younger children.

In the late 1980s while working as the child psychiatrist for a group of severely, behaviorally and emotionally troubled children in a special educational and treatment setting, I decided to do a an intensive clinical study of the most problematic and crisis prone of the youngsters enrolled in that program.[22, 23] These children and adolescents were admitted to the program because they were too unmanageable in their community schools. The majority of the children carried diagnoses of ADHD, conduct disorder, and the like. The children, who were known to experience psychotic phenomena such as hallucinations and delusions, were considered to suffer from schizophrenia. Bipolar disorder was rarely, if ever, considered a diagnosis in any of these children as per their records, even though most of these children had received psychiatric treatment—often for years—before enrollment in that program.

My comprehensive evaluation of these children, which extended over a period of approximately six months in most cases, included, among others, full history gathering from the children and parents (including informal evaluation of the parents), reviewing all past clinical and school records that could be obtained, observing the children daily when they attended school, formal and informal ongoing consultation and discussions with all therapists and teachers involved with the children, frequent follow up interviews to asses their functioning, progress, and response to treatment, as well as observations and obtaining relevant information during crisis interventions—a common occurrence with these children. How these evaluations were conducted is described in more detail in the two papers that resulted from these efforts.[22, 23] Since then, I have recommended such detailed evaluations and ongoing observations as necessary to diagnose bipolar disorder in children (often, not an easy undertaking in today's profit driven and fragmented clinical environment).

As a result of the above mentioned evaluations some surprising and shocking facts became evident. Of the twelve adolescents studied, eight were found to be definitely suffering from bipolar disorder, which, until then, had been misdiagnosed as ADHD and conduct disorder. Of the remaining four youngsters, three were exhibiting features highly suggestive of bipolar disorder, but they did not seem to satisfy the criteria for it as published in the official diagnostic manual at that time.[2] The fact that most (almost all) of these adolescents were suffering from bipolar disorder, which had gone unrecognized and misdiagnosed until then, was shocking indeed.

Even more amazing, were the findings on the group of pre-pubertal (younger) group of children studied. All five of the children of that group were found to suffer from bipolar disorder. None of these children had previously been diagnosed as suffering from this disorder. ADHD, and oppositional defiant disorder were the main diagnoses considered for these children in the past. Psychiatrists, who did past evaluations, diagnosed major depression in two children, atypical psychosis in two children, and schizophrenia in one child. One child was even considered to have narcissistic personality disorder (a diagnosis which is totally inappropriate in such young children, but which points to the clinicians' difficulty in understanding what is wrong with such children). However, in spite of such varying diagnostic manifestations appearing in these children from time to time, no one had given any consideration to the possibility that the children may be suffering from bipolar disorder. This omission or mistake appeared to be due to the fact that psychiatrists and other clinicians had little awareness that this illness could commonly occur in pre-pubertal children. As mentioned before, the common wisdom was, and still is, that bipolar disorder is an extreme rarity in pre-pubertal children.

Some important patterns became evident in reviewing the past history and records of the adolescents and younger children. **Most of these youngsters received a diagnosis of ADHD when they were in their early elementary school years.** As they became older, conduct disorder was added or replaced ADHD as the main diagnosis. One adolescent had received diagnoses of schizophrenia, and schizoaffective disorder. Various types of depression were noted in several of these youngsters, at times. Almost all these youngsters had experienced troublesome suicidal thoughts or urges at one time or another. Two of the adolescents had a history of wrist slashing. Two of the adolescents had even attempted suicide by hanging. However, none of the psychiatrists or other clinicians who evaluated or treated these children at various times in their lives, seemed to have looked at the total picture of their life time history and symptomatology, which would have made it clear (if they had awareness of this illness in children) that they suffered from bipolar disorder. Apart from the fact that, in the 1980's psychiatrists had very little awareness as to how common bipolar disorder was in children, other factors that contributed to the problem being unrecognized and which are also pertinent today, will be elaborated in the coming chapters.

About ten years back, I had the opportunity to treat a group of adolescents and younger children in an inpatient unit.[24] I took the opportunity to study the adolescents and children admitted to that unit during a six month period, using the same methodology of comprehensive evaluation, but extending over a shorter period of observation (since most of these youngsters were discharged from the unit within a month or so, if not earlier, after admission). I wanted to know how frequent bipolar disorder was in a group of children admitted to such an inpatient unit, as I had become convinced from my previous experience and studies, that the rate would be quite high, and that the frequency of past misdiagnosis would also be quite high. A total of 57 youngsters were admitted to the unit during the six-month period of the study. They included 44 adolescents and 13 younger (below 13 years of age) children. Findings similar to the ones mentioned before emerged as a result of this study also. Fourteen of the youngsters clearly met the official criteria [2] for bipolar disorder. An additional fifteen of the youngsters had enough signs and symptoms of the illness that they were considered "very likely" to be suffering from this illness.[24] Because of the short duration of their stay, it was not possible to rule out bipolar disorder in an additional fourteen of these children. It was quite clear that bipolar disorder was very common—if not the most common—diagnostic entity in hospitalized children—at least in such acute care units. Similar to the observation in the previously mentioned studies, it was clear that this illness had been recognized in very few of these children during their previous evaluations or hospitalizations. **ADHD, oppositional defiant disorder, conduct disorder, and occasional mention of depression, were the common diagnoses given to them previously.**

Another striking finding that emerged from this study was that **most children who suffered from psychotic phenomena such as hallucinations and delusions were found to have bipolar disorder rather than schizophrenia.** The common tendency has always been to diagnose schizophrenia or to give an indeterminate diagnosis of psychotic disorder not otherwise specified when phenomena such as hallucinations and delusions occurred.[2] Seldom is bipolar disorder considered a strong possibility in such children. However, in reality, **bipolar disorder may be the most common cause for such phenomena occurring in children**. A finding that emerged from this study that may be of great interest to people involved with the juvenile justice system is that thirteen, of the seventeen youngsters who were remanded to the unit by the courts, were found to be either definitely, or very likely suffering from bipolar disorder, [24] pointing to the strong possibility that **bipolar disorder may be the most common problem of troubled youngsters in the juvenile justice system.** The implications of such findings are discussed in more detail in the coming chapters.

During the past three years I have had the opportunity to evaluate and treat a great number of adolescents and children, who had a history of severe behavioral and emotional difficulties and who failed to respond to treatment and other interventions, that necessitated their enrollment in a special program for such difficult to treat youngsters. My evaluations of these youngsters have made it abundantly clear to me, once again, that **bipolar disorder continues to be the most common diagnostic entity** among seriously troubled and dysfunctional children, and that the tendency to misdiagnose bipolar disorder as ADHD and conduct disorder is still extremely prevalent.

My clinical experience of the past few decades, the studies mentioned above which I conducted, survey of the present literature on mental illness and problem behavior in children, and reports on related matters that appear in the lay press, etc., have made it clear to me that **bipolar disorder is occurring in epidemic proportions among our troubled youngsters, but is not recognized for what it is.** Because the illness goes undetected by professionals to such an astonishing degree, it is not receiving the urgent attention it deserves as a serious clinical, public health, and social problem. Though there has been a bit more awareness among child psychiatrists that this illness is more common in adolescents, and perhaps in younger children also, than was believed to be true in the past, the extent and depth of such awareness is woefully inadequate. Even the pronouncements from some of our reputed centers exhibit an ambivalence and lack of clarity in dealing with the subject of bipolar disorder in children.

As some senior clinicians and researchers are slowly becoming more aware that this illness is extremely widespread in children than they ever thought it was—but is still being misdiagnosed widely-, it appears, they are facing a dilemma. They appear to be unsure of how to own up to, and make amends for, the past mistake of not recognizing the extremely high prevalence of bipolar disorder in children–a lack of awareness that permeated the whole field of American Psychiatry for generations and continues even today. Such ignorance regarding this illness, obviously, also permeated many past and ongoing research efforts dealing with the problems of ADHD, conduct disorder, depression, etc., as many such research subjects may have been actually suffering from bipolar disorder instead of the problems they were mistakenly diagnosed with. **A great deal of research conclusions arrived upon regarding ADHD, conduct disorder, childhood depression, etc., may not be valid because of the mistake of bipolar subjects mistakenly included in such studies.**

The whole field of child psychiatry may have to do some soul searching to come to terms with such past mistakes, so that mistakes of this nature could be avoided in the future. The tendency of some clinicians and researchers to continue to diagnose, bipolar disorder co-morbid with ADHD, conduct disorder, etc., appear to be because of their inability to come to terms with such past mistakes. **The time has come for everyone to acknowledge the past mistakes and make a fresh start in coming to terms with the issue of bipolar disorder in children.**

There is urgent need for great deal of clarity to be brought to the issue of misdiagnosis of this disorder and for awareness as to how widespread the illness is in children. These issues require urgent attention because of the devastating personal and social effects such lack of awareness continues to exact—a situation that will only get worse, unless we, as a society, address the seriousness of the problem urgently.

Not many controlled studies have been done with large samples of children to ascertain the prevalence and manifestations of this illness in children. Some people may use this fact to deny that this illness is widespread in children. Before large controlled studies could be done, several conditions have to occur, however. To start with, people in decision making capacities and in allotting funding for such studies have to develop awareness that bipolar disorder in children is a serious, highly prevalent problem worthy of such large scale efforts. The criteria to diagnose bipolar disorder, for such study purposes have to be agreed upon. At present the criteria to diagnose bipolar disorder in children are not clearly delineated in official diagnostic manuals.[2] There has been widespread criticism that the criteria given in the diagnostic manuals are not even adequate to effectively diagnose bipolar disorders in adults, especially that the atypical and other common forms of the illness are not covered adequately. The concept of bipolar spectrum disorders [6,11] in adults, presently of great interest in the field, points to the growing awareness that bipolar disorders are a group of disorders with many common features for the group as a whole, but also having unique features specific to particular subgroups. This appears to be true in children also. There is a need to reach some consensus as to the usual manifestations of bipolar disorder in children (and adults). Before large-scale research studies can be undertaken, there is a need for a large cadre of clinician researchers, who will be capable of using such criteria arrived upon by consensus, to conduct studies to clarify issues related to the prevalence of this disorder and further refine diagnostic criteria, treatment efficacy, etc. At present, most large-scale research studies in child psychiatry are conducted using trainees, to interview participants in research and arrive upon diagnoses and other conclusions. Since, even senior clinicians very often misdiagnose this illness as other problems, the time has not yet come to depend on trainees to do the core ingredients of such research reliably. So also, **bipolar disorder cannot be diagnosed or ruled out by one or two interviews, in many, if not most children** (the method used in most large-scale studies). **Prolonged periods of repeated observations by knowledgeable and experienced clinicians are needed to confirm or rule out this illness in many children** (sometimes even extending for a period of one or more years). Presently there is no substitute to a highly experienced child psychiatrist (preferably the one who is treating the child), observing and evaluating the children carefully over a period of months or even years, to properly identify this illness in a reliable manner.

Clinicians, who have sufficient training and experience in child psychiatry, can use publications such as this to educate and guide them in their clinical work with such children, so that they will become experts in detecting and diagnosing bipolar disorder in children. This will also make them aware of how prevalent this illness is in children and how unrecognized it is. Only when a cadre of such competent clinician-researchers become available can large-scale research studies on bipolar disorder in children be conducted in a valid and reliable manner.

CHAPTER II

WHY IS THE PROBLEM UNRECOGNIZED?

It is common knowledge in American Psychiatry today, that until a decade or so back schizophrenia was vastly over diagnosed and manic-depressive Illness under-diagnosed in the United States. Though the situation has improved in the past decade, it is still very common to see psychiatric patients, who have spent even the greater part of their lives in psychiatric hospitals and other treatment settings, carrying a diagnosis of schizophrenia, but actually suffering from bipolar disorder. Even, when meeting many such patients for the first time, it would become quite clear to most knowledgeable psychiatrists that these patients have been misdiagnosed as schizophrenic, and that the bipolar disorder they suffer from has been misunderstood as schizophrenia. **Any psychiatrist who takes the time and effort, to obtain and review the past records of these unfortunate people** (most psychiatrists are not inclined to do so however today, because of time pressures, lack of monetary returns for the effort, lack of appropriate support staff in clinics, and other related problems) **can readily confirm the fact that they have been misdiagnosed as schizophrenic, when bipolar disorder or schizoaffective disorder–bipolar type[2] would be the appropriate diagnosis.** Such misdiagnosis of bipolar disorder as schizophrenia is not the only major problem of misdiagnosis however.

There has been widespread misdiagnosis of bipolar disorder, as borderline personality disorder (an overused and abused diagnosis in American Psychiatry, indicating the lack of understanding of clinicians as to the manifestations bipolar disorder), **or as other personality disorders,**

13

which results in erroneous treatment of such people not only clinically, but by the justice system and society as well. A diagnosis of personality disorder implies that the problem is due to character or personality defect and that such people are fully capable of changing their behavior. They are hence considered fully culpable for their actions. However, **the truth, more often than not is that, these people so misdiagnosed are actually suffering from bipolar disorder—a genetic illness, rather than any character defect.** Their problems are almost entirely due to the faulty genes or D.N.A. and related biochemistry they have inherited which control their brain function–a problem beyond their control. Such faulty brain chemistry and functioning that give rise to bipolar disorder, condemn them to a life of suffering and misunderstanding by others–even the professional who are there to help them.

It is not unusual to see vast numbers of people suffering from bipolar disorder incarcerated in jails, misdiagnosed with diagnoses such as antisocial or other personality disorders. People so misunderstood, abound in our substance abuse treatment settings also, where the bipolar disorder they suffer from and makes them vulnerable addiction to substances goes unrecognized, with the result that they continue to be dysfunctional and their chances for recovery from addiction severely compromised.

The fact that bipolar disorder is still under diagnosed and often misdiagnosed as unipolar depression and treated inappropriately with antidepressants only, was also pointed out even recently.[15] It is no wonder that, if misdiagnosis of bipolar disorder is still so prevalent in adults, the problem of misdiagnosis is even worse in children, since this illness has been considered an extreme rarity in children, to start with.

The belief that this disorder is extremely rare in children was conventional wisdom, and many, if not most clinicians and authorities in the field of child psychiatry perpetuated this myth. I remember, how in the mid 1980s, a senior academic who was conducting a course for prospective candidates for the American Board Examination in Child Psychiatry, emphasizing that the examiners would be very understanding and in general would try to help the candidates pass the examination, unless they–the candidates—blurted out "blunders," such as, stating that a pre-pubertal child they had interviewed or whose interview they had observed on video may be suffering from bipolar disorder. What this expert child psychiatrist was conveying to the candidates was that, bipolar disorder was such a rarity in children, that one was risking sure failure in the examination, if one ventured that it was worthy of being considered as a serious differential diagnosis in children. The situation has not changed much since then. **Even experienced child psychiatrists in supervisory positions convey such misinformation to trainees, and they in turn continue to perpetuate this myth throughout their career.**

Common Causes for Misdiagnosis in Children

The Most Common Mistake: over diagnosis of ADHD

American child psychiatry has suffered from the overemphasis and over diagnosis of ADHD. Other disruptive behavior disorders[2] such as conduct disorder and oppositional defiant disorder are also commonly and erroneously diagnosed when the children are actually suffering from bipolar disorder or one of its variants. This tendency to over-diagnose ADHD and the related disruptive behavior disorders mentioned above has gone on for the past half century or more in the U.S. It has prevented the clinicians from considering other relevant diagnoses, when the child's problems indicate that some thing other than such disorders might be the reason for the child's problems.[22,23,24] **Generations of clinicians have been trained under the erroneous notion that ADHD, conduct disorder, etc., are the most common problems in children who exhibit behavior problems, and that bipolar disorder is an extreme rarity in children.** Because of this, any child who is overactive, impulsive, quick to anger, a serious discipline problem, etc., is almost always diagnosed with ADHD, with an additional sprinkling of oppositional defiant disorder or conduct disorder added in the older children. Invariably, most of these children will receive prolonged periods of treatment with stimulants (such as Ritalin and Dexedrine) and an assortment of psychotherapeutic attempts, with little lasting or consistent benefit. Most of the seriously troubled children will not respond in any consistent manner to these treatments and will be shuttled from one treatment setting to another—even inpatient facilities and residential treatment centers—repeatedly, with little lasting benefit. The diagnostic understanding will continue to be ADHD and the other disruptive disorders, as clinicians often do not know what else could be the reason for the child's non-responding and waxing and waning problems. **The pervasive thinking in the field of child psychiatry—explaining away most overactive, impulsive, and troublesome behavior as ADHD, conduct disorder, etc., only-, blind the clinicians from recognizing the true nature of these children's problems**—which more often than not, on careful scrutiny, will turn out to be bipolar disorder. [22,23,24]

The Issue of Co-morbidity with ADHD

Another reason for not properly understanding the problems of such children is that, once ADHD is entertained as the diagnosis, clinicians are very reluctant to let go of it and consider another more relevant and serious illness, such as bipolar disorder, even when it becomes clear that ADHD or other disruptive disorders cannot explain the children's problems. For example, a child diagnosed as having ADHD may exhibit signs of major depression, serious and persistent conduct problems, pathological elation or excitation (even frank manic features at times), other signs of mood and anxiety disorders, even hallucinations (if carefully observed and questioned by a knowledgeable person) and delusional beliefs. These manifestations should alert the clinician that something more sinister than ADHD, conduct disorder, etc., is the reason for these manifestations. Instead the manner in which our clinicians are taught to approach such problems, make them, either ignorant of such considerations altogether or diagnose each aspect of problem behavior or symptomatology as an additional diagnosis superimposed on ADHD. For example, a child initially diagnosed as having ADHD may develop severe depression, in which case the clinicians add major depression or dysthymia[2] to the ADHD diagnosis—the depression, considered as occurring "co-morbid" with ADHD.

Because of such illogical thinking, one frequently sees children carrying multiple diagnoses such as, ADHD co-morbid with depression, conduct disorder, oppositional defiant disorder, anxiety disorder, obsessive-compulsive disorder, etc. Children so diagnosed with multiple co-morbid problems are treated with combinations of medicines by psychiatrists each medicine supposedly aiming at each co-morbid condition. The usual pattern is: one or more stimulant medicines–mainly Ritalin or Dexedrine that they consider as mandatory treatment for the ADHD—and additional medicines to address each co-morbid condition.

In reality, however, **a careful examination of the child's problems, in many cases, would lead to the diagnosis of one all-encompassing condition such as bipolar disorder**. For example, the co-occurrence of features of ADHD along with signs of severe conduct disorder and depression in a waxing and waning manner points to bipolar disorder being the crucial and central problem of children thus affected. Features of bipolar disorder will explain symptoms of ADHD, conduct disorder, oppositional defiant disorder, recurrent or admixture of depression, and even periodic occurrence of symptoms such as hallucinations and delusions. **Features of many anxiety disorders—even obsessive-compulsive disorder-, and eating disorders occur in many bipolar children.** Such manifestations are in keeping with the evolving concept of "bipolar spectrum disorders" [6,19] in adult psychiatric literature.

Astonishingly, clinicians even diagnose ADHD co-morbid with bipolar disorder. **Once a child is found to suffer from bipolar disorder there is little reason to consider a diagnosis of ADHD along with it as an additional diagnosis**, as all the manifestations of ADHD, such as hyperactivity, impulsivity, inability to remain focused on school work, being disruptive, etc., are common symptoms of manic, hypomanic, or mixed manifestations of bipolar disorder.[2] Diagnosing mania or hypomania of bipolar disorder, as being co-morbid with ADHD is somewhat similar to saying that a person suffers from schizophrenia but also has a co-morbid delusional disorder, or that someone suffers from major depressive disorder, but also has a co-morbid sleep disorder.

One does not diagnose an adult who is in manic state with his thought and attention jumping from one subject to another in rapid succession and who is overactive and disruptive to his environment–among the classical features of mania-, as suffering from mania or bipolar disorder and ADHD. Yet, with children, any child who is hyperactive or impulsive today is automatically given a diagnosis of ADHD, and additional features or problems exhibited by the child are considered additional diagnoses or illnesses. So, in toady's psychiatric reports one commonly comes across ADHD co-morbid with depression, conduct disorder, psychotic disorder, etc. In actuality, the child, more often than not, may be suffering from bipolar disorder, which would encompass all the features in the diagnostic entities mentioned above. The tendency to diagnose multiple diagnostic conditions as co-morbid with ADHD is a bit like the story of the "Blind Men and the Elephant," in which each blind man tries to feel out with his hand what an elephant looks like and ends up mistaking the shape of the particular part of the elephant each one touches, to be the shape of the elephant (the one who happens to handle the ears imagining the elephant looks like a large leaf, the one who examined the leg, that the elephant is shaped like a pillar and so on), but missing the total picture: the elephant.

The, Once ADHD Always ADHD Thinking

Once ADHD is diagnosed in a child (rightly or wrongly) and the child enters treatment for this condition, in most problematic cases, sooner or later, the child will be prescribed treatment with a stimulant medication such as Ritalin (methylphenidate) or Dexedrine (dextroamphetamine). Once the child is placed on such stimulant medications, even if the problems fail to improve—or even worsen-, doctors fail to stop treatment with such medicines and will usually add on other medicines, thinking they are treating ADHD and additional "co-morbid conditions." In actuality, they may have misdiagnosed the problem, and the medicines, instead of being helpful, may even be making the condition worse or may be acting against each other nullifying their effects. **This often occurs because of the erroneous notion that hyperactivity, impulsivity, and poor concentration capacity mean ADHD—and ADHD only, and whatever other features may be present are due to additional co-morbid conditions.** Based on such erroneous thinking, psychiatrists prescribe Ritalin or another stimulant to address ADHD, and additional medicines to treat the so-called co-morbid conditions. This is why it is common to see children being treated and discharged from even major teaching centers today on a combination of Ritalin and a variety of other medicines such as neuroleptics, mood regulators (Depakote, lithium, etc.), and antidepressants. In my experience, children, more often than not, do poorly on such combinations, as their problems are often due to bipolar disorder, and such combinations of medicines, instead of helping, more or less act against each other and nullify their effects. They may even worsen the condition of the children and expose them unnecessarily to the toxicity of multiple medicines. Ritalin and other stimulants either do not help the bipolar illness or in some cases may even make it worse, especially if the child is in a manic or mixed phase of the illness. Parents often state, "It made him worse, he was climbing the walls with it." Moreover, such incongruous combinations of medicines suggest that the clinician is not knowledgeable enough to evaluate the child's complex symptomatology, and hence, is likely to have difficulty charting out a cohesive and effective treatment approach.

The Ritalin-effect Dilemma

Another issue that confounds the thinking of psychiatrists and others, often, is the effect medicines such as Ritalin have on children. These medicines, which are basically stimulants, are known to improve the capacity of people to concentrate for a few hours when they are taken. Ritalin and other stimulant medicines have been used or abused by college students in many countries when they were easily available, to keep awake at night and cram for examinations. They are known to improve the attention and concentration capacities of many children diagnosed as having ADHD, for a few hours after each dose. They may also make the children quieter and less hyperactive for the same short period. At times these medicines make the children behave in a withdrawn and listless manner while under their effect–a state the parents find distressing. However, there is little evidence whether these medicines will have much positive effect in the long run on their academic achievement and behavior and on their functioning when they reach adulthood.

In my experience, **the severely troubled of the hyperactive and impulsive children—a group that would contain many bipolar children, though not recognized as such-, do not consistently do well on Ritalin or other stimulants.** More often, the drug may have an inconsistent effect: at times appearing to have some beneficial effect (probably when the children are in a depressive phase or in a period of remission of the bipolar illness), at other times having no discernible benefit, and at times their problems appearing to be even worse while taking these medicines. The high probability, of medicines such as Ritalin and Dexedrine worsening the behavior of children who suffer from bipolar disorder is quite understandable, as stimulants such as these can make mania or hypomania worsen, or may even induce such states in children prone to develop such states. **Most children who suffer from bipolar disorder exhibit a pattern of periodic worsening while being maintained on the same dose of stimulant medicines such as Ritalin or Dexedrine, pointing to the strong possibility that the problem is related to bipolar disorder rather than ADHD.** Unfortunately, many doctors fail to recognize this and usually increase the dose of the stimulants more and more, most likely worsening the situation, or add other medicines–again, an unwise move, as the medicines often counteract each other or worsen the toxic effects of each other.

Such sorry state of affairs can go on for many years, with periodic worsening of the children's condition, need for hospitalizations, etc., until the child becomes an adult, by which time, usually, he or she may have dropped out of high school, and may have become a highly dysfunctional or obviously mentally ill adult. **They often end up in jails or become homeless, with the true nature of their problem–bipolar disorder-not recognized or treated.** Today, one finds among the ranks of the chronically mentally ill adults, the homeless, and in our prison populations many who were misunderstood and mistreated thus when they were children. One comes across many adults who suffer from bipolar disorder today, who give a history of having been diagnosed with ADHD (erroneously) when they were children and treated with medicines such as Ritalin for years.

The Fragmented Treatment and Unknown Histories of Children

Another reason why psychiatrists and clinicians have not become competent in identifying bipolar disorder in children is the fragmentation in the treatment and care of seriously troubled children. Often, it is extremely difficult (and not very remunerative) for psychiatrists in private office practice to carry these children in treatment, year after year, as the children's condition would require, because of the inordinate amount of time and effort needed to properly deal with their problems. The children are often crisis prone, extremely uncooperative, and aggressive, which causes great deal of stress for the doctors treating such children and disruptive to the smooth running of an office practice. Most of these children's treatment would not go on in a smooth, predictable manner. More often than not, there are frequent, broken appointments, uncooperative behavior, crisis after crisis of behavioral and symptom worsening, major disciplinary problems at home and school, suspensions from school, legal problems, etc., requiring a great deal of effort and interventions from the psychiatrist. Almost always, the monetary compensation for such efforts is inadequate–especially in today's managed care environment. The psychiatrists will find that, they cannot have a smooth running office practice if they have many such children in their case load, because the crisis proneness of the children interfere with the psychiatrist's capacity to provide care for other patients who expect predictable appointment schedule, uninterrupted attention from the psychiatrist, etc. Hence, after an initial period of treatment attempts, the more problematic of such children, sooner or later, will be transferred to a clinic setting where there are psychiatrists, trainees, and other clinicians available to help address the varied needs of these children, as their situation demands from time to time. Thus, most of these children are treated in not-for-profit community mental health clinics or child psychiatry clinics attached to teaching hospitals where most of the treatment is done by doctors training to become psychiatrists (Residents), other trainees, or other early-career mental health professionals.

Unfortunately, in most clinics their treatment gets transferred from staff member to staff member,—or even worse, the children are transferred from clinic to clinic, with periodic in-patient hospitalizations, and even admissions to residential treatment centers, in a chaotic and repetitive manner. This results in no one really having a comprehensive understanding of the nature of these children's symptomatology on a continuum-a requirement for properly identifying bipolar disorder in children.[22,23,24] As the children get transferred from clinician-to-clinician or facility-to-facility, they receive a variety of poorly thought out diagnoses and treatment attempts—often the clinicians responsible for their care not knowing what the symptomatology or problems were at various times in the past and how and why various professionals arrived at various conclusions in the past. The result is that the total picture of a child's problems, symptomatology, and history that may point to bipolar disorder is not recognized, and the child ends up being misdiagnosed and inappropriately treated.

Lack of Guidelines for Diagnosing Bipolar Disorder in Children

Probably, because of the erroneous notion that bipolar disorder is rare in children, the criteria for diagnosing this disorder in children have not been adequately addressed in psychiatric literature–even in D.S.M.

IV.[2] This makes it more difficult for clinicians to suspect and diagnose this disorder in children. Moreover, the criteria given in D.S.M. IV[2] are based on observations with adult patients who suffer from, more or less, classical forms of the illness. Experienced clinicians and researchers in the field of bipolar disorder have been increasingly vocal about how such criteria are even inadequate in identifying many adults who suffer from the various forms of this illness. [1, 11, 15, 19, 32] The increasing numbers of papers published and seminars held on "Bipolar Spectrum Disorders" in adults today, also attest to this fact.[1,6] Frequently, many of the adults may have been exhibiting features of bipolar disorder for quite some time—even years, if not from their childhood—until the full blown episodes manifest in a manner that most psychiatrists recognize to be bipolar disorder. In some cases, the manifestations of the illness may appear abruptly and in dramatic form (this happens usually in classical bipolar disorder), as an episode of acute mania or depression, with or without a claer precipitant.

When one closely examines the histories of many manic-depressive adults, it would appear that their illness had been manifesting in subtle and not so subtle forms for quite some time before it was recognized for what it is. Many of these adults have a history of significant emotional or behavioral problems starting at a young age—often from adolescence if not earlier. These problems usually would have been misunderstood and given diagnoses such as ADHD, or oppositional defiant disorder, conduct disorder, depressive disorder NOS[2], etc. Some youngsters who may have been hospitalized may have received diagnoses such as depression or psychotic disorder NOS[2] or a mixture of the above mentioned type of diagnoses, depending on who evaluated them, and when, and under what circumstances.

The points mentioned above and related observations have made it clear to psychiatrists seriously interested in the field of bipolar disorder in children and adults, that bipolar disorder, especially in its atypical forms, very often starts manifesting in childhood or adolescence, but is seldom recognized for what it is. This state of affairs with regard to diagnosis may not fully change until reliable biological tests become available to diagnose this illness accurately. However, in most cases, the disorder could be strongly suspected, and later diagnosed with almost sure certainty, even in young children, if clinicians maintain a strong awareness as to how common this disorder is in children and are knowledgeable of its varied manifestations in them. They also have to have the commitment, patience, and time required to undertake such a venture.

Eager to Diagnose Depression but Bipolar not a Consideration

When we look through the psychiatric evaluation reports and literature in children there is a great deal of mention of depression as a major problem but very little mention of bipolar disorder. It is very common to see diagnoses such as depressive disorder NOS, dysthymia, and even major depression recurrent [2] among the diagnoses in many children's psychiatric reports, with the almost ever present ADHD, oppositional defiant disorder and conduct disorder liberally sprinkled along with it. The tendency to diagnose depression but failure to see the total picture of bipolar disorder, as a very prevalent form of misdiagnosis and under-diagnosis in adults, has been pointed out even recently.[15] Whenever one sees such combinations of diagnoses of depression and disruptive disorders such as ADHD or conduct disorder and the like, one has to be alert to the strong possibility that bipolar disorder may be the actual problem but may be going unrecognized. Common sense itself would tell us that a child who is suffering from serious depression is unlikely to have the energy and drive to engage in the type of aggressive, impulsive, fun seeking, and antisocial activities that are often described in the case histories of such children, if their problem is only depression. When a child is described as meriting a diagnosis of depression of one type or another, at one time or another, by one or more clinicians, and the child has also been described as having severe behavior problems meriting diagnoses of ADHD or oppositional defiant disorder or conduct disorder, and the like, either simultaneously with depression, or on separate occasions, it is essential that a healthy suspicion be maintained that the totality of the problem may be bipolar disorder. [22,23,24] In this context, based on my experience with such problems, I suggest that clinicians keep in mind the following formula:

Depression+ADHD and/or Oppositional defiant disorder, or Conduct disorder=? Bipolar disorder

Reluctance to Diagnose Bipolar Disorder

Bipolar disorder(s), being a serious mental disorder or a group of related disorders with varying intensities and complexities in their manifestations, with not-very-good or poor prognosis in many cases (given today's limited remedies available), it is understandable and wise that clinicians exercise great caution in arriving at such a diagnosis. However, when the diagnosis is definitely or strongly evident, avoiding such consideration can only make matters worse. There are several obvious and not so obvious reasons why clinicians fail to make such a diagnosis even when the evidence for it is strong. The first and foremost, as mentioned before, is the lack of awareness of the manner in, and frequency with which this illness occurs in children. Another reason is the stigma attached to such a diagnosis and the negative, fearful reaction such a diagnosis provokes in parents, children,—and even the colleagues of clinicians who make such diagnosis.

Psychiatrists and other clinicians are often hesitant and unwilling to face such negative reactions and the resulting criticism that he or she is misdiagnosing children as suffering from this serious—and in the opinion of the critics a very rare–illness, when the children's problems are only ADHD or "behavioral" in their opinion. Many psychiatrists would rather avoid such controversial situations and opt for diagnostic terms that are more acceptable in child psychiatry–ADHD being the easiest choice in such situations and the most acceptable "politically."

Since bipolar disorder has been historically under-diagnosed in children, psychiatrists are ill equipped to deal with the plethora of reactions such a diagnosis invariably elicits from multiple sources. There is little in the literature or what they can learn from senior clinicians, as to how to deal with the reactions set in motion by their arriving on such a diagnosis. In this context, it is worth mentioning that most child psychiatric clinics are now headed by non-medical personnel, and they are even more unfamiliar with the diagnosis and management of illnesses such as bipolar disorder in children (not surprising, since most child psychiatrists also consider the illness to be a rarity) and very uncomfortable dealing with such diagnoses and children who are affected by such illnesses.

In general, many non-medical professionals subscribe to the theory that children's problems are primarily, if not entirely, reactions to environmental problems or due to faulty attitudes of parents, and as such, are to be addressed primarily by psychotherapy—often psychoanalytically oriented psychotherapy, family therapy, etc. **This produces an atmosphere in these clinics that is not conducive to honest discourse on diagnostic and related clinical issues, with a subsequent tendency by psychiatrists to under-diagnose bipolar disorder, to stay out of the controversy.** (The psychiatrists, for reasons mentioned before, are prone, not to detect bipolar disorder when it exists, to start with.) Non-medical leaders of these clinics face an additional disincentive not to recognize the problem of extremely high prevalence of bipolar disorder in their clientele. If the children's problems are recognized as bipolar disorder, then the treatment emphasis moves primarily from the realm of psychotherapy, to psychiatric management, and pharmacotherapy for the illness becomes the crucial aspect of such children's treatment. Such a shift in emphasis and leadership of treatment to the psychiatrist is not acceptable in many clinics. Such clinics and their leadership operate on the notion that the psychotherapist is the primary care giver and decision maker. This is in part because of the belief that children's problems are mostly "behavioral" or "reactive" in nature, and hence psychotherapy is the most important aspect of any child's treatment. The child psychiatrist is only considered a consultant to provide prescriptions to keep some problems in check, where as psychotherapy provided by therapists are considered the primary, crucial, and curative form of treatment for children. These facts are well known to all who have experience with the "politics" of how today's clinics function, but seldom articulated because of the obvious unease–even catastrophic effects on ones professional and financial well being—such opinions provoke. However, **when dealing with serious illnesses such as bipolar disorder in children, one cannot avoid facing facts, how unpleasant or "politically incorrect" they may be, as doing otherwise will be a disservice to the children and their families,—a grave, moral and ethical lapse.**

In such clinics there is also the concern that if the problem is bipolar disorder—which is due to the action of faulty genes and biochemistry, more than anything else-, requiring that these children and families participate in weekly psychotherapy or family therapy sessions month after month–even year after year—becomes unreasonable and difficult to justify. This is especially so, if the parents and children object to it or become uninterested and uncooperative with such measures, as it often happens in such situations. Such lack of interest often occurs, as the children and parents find participation in such sessions indefinitely, not very useful in addressing their primary problem: bipolar disorder and its ill effects on them. This occurs, especially, when the therapists loose track of the fact that the child and family are there because of a biological illness that is the root cause of the child's disturbed behavior and emotional turmoil. In today's managed care environment, insurance companies also balk at weekly open-ended psychotherapy sessions for children with such diagnoses. Such predicaments are not acceptable to the administration of many of the clinics, for economic reasons also, as weekly psychotherapy sessions generate badly needed income for the clinics.

Often many of these clinics have a rule that the children have to be seen weekly by the psychotherapist as long as they are enrolled in the clinic, or otherwise they cannot continue to receive services from the clinic (which means they cannot continue to see the psychiatrist who has been providing pharmacotherapy and related services for them). This results in the children and family dropping out of treatment or being unhappy and mistrusting of the whole treatment process and the motives of the professionals. Unfortunately, many bipolar children and adults are victimized one way or another by the "system" in these manners throughout their lives–by the very professionals who are supposed to help them and do what is right for them.

A common sense, flexible approach, in which the child's illness and well being are kept as central issues, and services are provided in a flexible manner relevant to the child's condition and need from time to time, is essential for the successful treatment of children who suffer from bipolar disorder.

Mistaking Bipolar Disorder in Adolescents for Borderline Personality Disorder

The concept of borderline personality disorder[2] has been a controversial one, even with adults. Unfortunately, in the United States, a great deal of speculative writing has gone on about the concept of "borderline personality," and many people have made a name for themselves based on such writings. Experts on bipolar disorder in adults, have expressed the opinion that many people diagnosed as suffering from borderline personality disorder, on closer scrutiny, would actually found to be suffering from bipolar disorder, instead.[1] There is a tendency to diagnose many people who are behaviorally and emotionally unstable (a hall mark of atypical forms of bipolar disorder) and difficult to treat, as having borderline personality. Conventional wisdom is that they require prolonged periods of psychoanalytically oriented psychotherapy to attain the personality growth they need to be delivered from their problems. The reality is that, most people so diagnosed fail to improve by psychotherapy alone because they actually are suffering from bipolar disorder[1], the manifestations of which are pretty much beyond their control—no matter how hard they try to improve their personality. Today, the term "borderline personality" has attained a pejorative connotation in the mental health field. Mental health professionals often use this term to describe a person who is difficult to treat, is emotionally unstable, volatile, unreasonably demanding, crisis prone, whose symptomatology varies widely, including experiencing and exhibiting hallucinations and delusions at times, etc. Clinicians erroneously believe that such people have the capacity to control their behavior and symptomatology if only they will adhere to their therapist's advice to attain "insight" and attain the personality growth they need–a "Catch 22" situation for the patient. The term "borderline" is used by professionals, often in a defensive manner also, to suggest that such people seldom get better unless they remain in intensive insight oriented therapy for a very long time (years) to attain the personality growth they need to move up from the "borderline" level—while keeping their emotions and behavior in control (which they cannot do because the bipolar illness they suffer from play havoc with their emotions, behavior, and lives). The inability of the patient to accomplish the unrealistic tasks the clinicians demand of them, is taken as an example of the patient's lack of motivation in getting better and not due to any faults in the clinicians' understanding and approach to the problem. **Unfortunately, not recognizing that many people diagnosed as "borderline" are actually suffering from bipolar disorder and not instituting treatment for bipolar disorder are, often, the main reasons why such people fail to improve at least to some degree.** This predicament in adult psychiatry also occurs to many adolescents who suffer from atypical forms of bipolar disorder. Adolescents who are emotionally and behaviorally unstable, crisis prone, indulge in gestures such as wrist slashing and taking overdoses when they are unhappy, upset, or angry, and who experience transient psychotic phenomena are often diagnosed erroneously as having borderline personality–or at least that is the term clinicians often use to describe them-, when, in actuality, they may be suffering from bipolar disorder. Often, mental health professionals insist that such adolescents should be treated primarily, or only by psychotherapeutic efforts, as they are considered to be suffering from a personality problem–and hence, need personality growth promoting psychotherapy as their primary or only modality of treatment. Many such adolescents actually suffer from bipolar disorder, and their illness will go unrecognized, at times all through their lives, as they get saddled with the erroneous diagnosis of borderline personality, from a young age, which will make clinicians view them with the same prejudice such a diagnostic term elicits when they become adults also.

Another unfortunate aspect of such misdiagnosis is that, they would also be found ineligible for financial and medical insurance benefits that they truly deserve from government or other agencies, because their problem is considered to be a personality disorder only (which implies that they choose that way of life) and not a serious mental illness. Since many if not most such adolescents grow up to be highly dysfunctional adults, incapable of earning a living for themselves, and the true nature of their illness which manifested in childhood or adolescence have not been properly diagnosed or documented, both the Social Security and the Welfare or Social Assistance systems reject their requests for assistance, if and when they apply for such benefits. Such predicaments increase the possibility of their becoming homeless and to their turning to a life of crime to support them-selves. This is also an example of the ways in which unrecognized bipolar disorder plays a crucial role in present day social turmoil. **The time has come for those in charge of diagnostic manuals and classifications in psychiatry, to re-evaluate the whole concept of borderline personality–a concept, which, in my opinion, hinders rather than helps in the proper understanding and treatment of mentally ill people today.**

Objection by Parents and Children to the Diagnosis of Bipolar Disorder

There are also factors related to the children and parents, which inhibit the identification and diagnosis of bipolar disorder in children. In general, most people do not want to believe or admit they are mentally ill—for reasons that are easy to understand and anyone can empathize with. This problem is perhaps most severe in bipolar disorder. Bipolar disorder is considered a mental illness (though in reality it is due to chemical abnormalities of the brain, and in this sense is not very different from many other "physical" diseases affecting the brain), which, especially in its manic, hypomanic or mixed phases, smothers the capacity of people suffering from it, from recognizing that they are ill. Adolescents vehemently oppose the idea of such an illness being the reason for their problems. Parents are afraid and very reluctant to accept such a diagnosis and explanation for their children's problems. They would prefer to believe that their son or daughter is "bad" or is being influenced by the "wrong crowd," rather than consider them to be affected by such an illness. Given the inadequate remedies for serious mental illnesses available today, the stigma attached to mental illness in society, and the fear and despondency such a diagnosis elicits, one cannot blame the parents or children for such resistance. Moreover, the children, as with adults who suffer from this illness, more often than not, will continue to lack insight that they are ill, as the illness–especially in its continuous and atypical forms—almost blends in with their very nature, which makes it difficult—if not impossible—for most sufferers to distinguish between how the illness makes them feel and behave and what they will be like if they were not affected by the illness. One cannot expect a person who is pathologically excited and in turmoil with mania or hypomania, to retain the self-observing capacity or insight that what he is experiencing and how he is behaving are abnormal and are the results of abnormal functioning of his brain. With children, the capacity for such self-awareness is even less. Many youngsters with bipolar disorder state, "This is me…this is how I was born." A great deal of experience and patience on the part of the psychiatrist in addressing such lack of insight in the child and parents, would be necessary to help them come to terms with these predicaments in the best way they can, so that they may cooperate with reasonable treatment measures. **Mental illnesses such as bipolar disorder are unique in this regard, as they change the observational capacities of the very organ (brain) that is the essential instrument for self-observation and awareness.**

Given these circumstances, it is no wonder that clinicians diagnose each phenomenon they observe in the child as a separate entity, rather than consider the diagnosis of bipolar disorder, which alone would explain the varying aspects of the child's problems. **In most cases it is easier for the psychiatrist to say that the child suffers from ADHD, even when it is clear that actually the problem is bipolar disorder. Many psychiatrists unfortunately prefer to take the easier route of rubber-stamping the diagnosis of ADHD until the child gets lost somewhere and is no more their concern. A combination of psychiatrists' lack of knowledge of bipolar disorder in children and their reluctance to face criticism or disapproval from colleagues, parents, the youngsters themselves, and others lie behind the failure to identify and diagnose bipolar disorder, when such diagnosis is really warranted.**

CHAPTER III

BIPOLAR DISORDER IN PRE-PUBERTAL CHILDREN

Though there is much that is common with the expression of bipolar disorder in children, compared to that in adolescents, there are also features that differ in their expression in one of these age groups compared to the other. Some psychiatrists, who can accurately identify bipolar disorder in adolescents, may have difficulty identifying the illness in younger children because of the manner in which the illness manifests in them. Because of this, the manifestations of the illness in these two age groups are discussed separately in this publication, while acknowledging that there is considerable overlap between the two. In this chapter the term child or children is used to refer to youngsters of pre-pubertal age.

Before we discuss the symptomatology of bipolar disorder in children, some clarification and caution are needed. Bipolar disorder—as in adults also—presents in classical, and non-classical or atypical forms in children. In the classical form of the illness, discrete episodes of mania occur with pathologically elated or euphoric mood, increased energy, over activity, over talkativeness, pressured speech, hyper-sexuality, decreased need for sleep, grandiose delusions, and at times hallucinations also. The manic episodes are interspersed with depressive episodes, with or without intervening periods of full remission or normality. On the other hand, the depressive episodes of manic-depressive illness, often presents with decreased energy, insomnia (which is upsetting to the sufferer, compared to the reduced need for sleep or refusal to sleep which occurs in mania) or hypersomnia (excessive sleep), decrease in verbal productivity, depressed mood (often, but not always), tendency for withdrawal, at times hallucinations and/or delusions (usually mood congruent), and a tendency for suicidal ruminations or urges (if the depression is severe). This form of bipolar disorder (the classical variety) is not very common in children, but when it occurs, most experienced clinicians should be able to detect it without much difficulty, as the features are very similar to the adult form of the illness. Of course, some allowance has to be given for minor modifications in the symptomatology because of the age of the child. For example, a feature such as the tendency to go on shopping sprees and ruin one's finances, which often occurs in the adult manic, manifests in children in its childhood equivalent of incessant and irrational demands for objects of pleasure such as toys, video games, expensive clothes, and other articles of interest to children, accompanied by severe tantrums and even violent behavior if there demands are not given into. Such children often indulge in stealing from the parents and others—even large sums of money-, and buy articles of interest to them indiscriminately and excessively. They often use money obtained thus, to buy and distribute toys, candy, and such other articles indiscriminately to their peers. Such behavior can even attain bizarre proportions in the manic child. Often, they make little attempt to hide such prohibited behavior from adults—a finding, which often helps distinguish such behavior induced by bipolar disorder, from that seen in children with conduct disorder.

A twelve-year-old-boy, who had been receiving stimulant medications for presumed ADHD for the past six years, from a major teaching hospital, had been exhibiting features indicative of bipolar disorder. During a period of worsening of symptomatology and behavior—which, in my opinion, was due to mania, he stole a few hundred dollars from his family. He denied taking the money, but during the next few days he frequently went out of the house and came back with an assortment of objects he had purchased, which included seven or eight large, flamboyant looking watches meant for adults. He took his grandmother's hand bag and brought it to the school and presented it to his teacher, as a gift, along with an assortment of canned foods he had been taking from home and hiding. His teacher had been in daily contact with his family about his behavior problems, but he appeared to be oblivious or unconcerned that she would immediately report such behavior to his family members. He had a long-standing history of sleeping poorly at night, remaining active and engaged in various inappropriate activities at night unconcerned he was disturbing the sleep of other family members. He was excessively and irrationally demanding, and a major discipline problem at home and school. He had been transferred from program to program and school to school through the years while being treated with stimulant medications and psychotherapy. All his problems worsened during the period mentioned above, when he stayed sleepless and overactive day and night, claiming to be superman and engaging in wild, "wrestling" moves he watched on T.V., that endangered his own safety and the safety of others.

Behavior and history such as those mentioned above cannot be explained by ADHD or conduct disorder. Such behavior and the accompanying symptomatology often attains an intensity in children with bipolar disorder that makes their management at home, school, and the out patient setting almost impossible.

The child mentioned above had gone through many such episodes in the past while being treated with stimulants, but his psychiatrists and other clinicians had failed to consider bipolar disorder as the cause for his disturbed behavior. He had continued to receive high doses of stimulant medicines such as Ritalin and Dexedrine year after year, because the notion that his problems were due to ADHD had not been reexamined in any competent manner during the years, even though he had been doing poorly and his behavior and symptomatology had been going through repeated periods of worsening to crisis proportions. This is also an example of the problem of the diagnosis of ADHD given to a child early in his life, remaining as a permanent diagnosis even after evidence mounts in later years that the problem is something else—most often bipolar disorder.

What we are mostly concerned in this section of bipolar disorder in pre-pubertal children, however, is the type of bipolar disorder that is more common during childhood—the one in which classical features of mania or depression do not occur in easily identifiable episodes, and in which, such features, if they occur, are often masked by more or less persistent behavioral and emotional problems. In such children the episodes of elation or excitability often do not reach the full manic intensity, but rather appear as a worsening of the behavior problems and intense emotionality which are part and parcel of the very nature of such children. Because of this, clinicians seldom recognize the bipolar nature of their problems. Often, features of elation and depression commingle in these children, giving them an emotionally over sensitive, unstable, and volatile quality. Instead of being elated and euphoric, these children are often highly excitable, irritable, and more than anything else, exhibit a tendency to be angry and aggressive—the frequent complaint that brings them to the psychiatrist. They are highly temperamental, and seldom pleasant and easygoing–at least not for long stretches of time. In such children, episodes of depression–if they ever occur in a discrete manner at all, are often not recognized by parents or clinicians because such depressive phases or episodes lack the full-blown features of major depression, clinicians are accustomed to seeing in adults. Such manifestations make the identification of the illness and differentiating it from "behavioral problems" or ADHD, quite difficult for most clinicians who are not fully familiar with the issue of bipolar disorder in children. Children, who suffer from such forms of bipolar disorder, generally do not experience significant periods of full remission of their problem behavior or symptomatology. More likely, there are periods of partial remission or improvement, followed by worsening. Such patterns of waxing-and-waning of the illness, make these children appear, as if they engage in bad behavior willfully–behavior which they are capable of controlling "if they want to." Adults interpret the frequent, inevitable occurrence of periods of worsening behavior in these children—especially the tendency for aggression, excitement, pathological anger, and often, over-activity and impulsivity as well–, to what they perceive as these children's lack of commitment to "being good." Clinicians usually think of such children as suffering from ADHD or oppositional defiant disorder or conduct disorder, and the like. Though the classical and atypical forms of the disorder vary in their presentation, they are not always mutually exclusive. The atypical form of bipolar disorder, in many ways, appear to be a variant of the classical type of the disorder, with the symptomatology expressing various gradations and admixtures of manic and depressive symptomatology in less than full blown intensity, but at the same time, existing as a chronic phenomenon in a waxing-and-waning manner without periods of full remission. The bipolar disorder such children suffer from is in many ways similar to the varieties of bipolar or related disorders increasingly discussed in literature on adult patients under the terms "bipolar spectrum disorders," "sub-threshold forms of bipolar disorder," etc.[1]

A child who suffers predominantly from the atypical form or forms of this illness, may, at times exhibit more classical features of mania or major depression with or without hallucinations or delusions. So also, a child who has exhibited classical mania or depression could exhibit the atypical features noted above, at times. This usually occurs when the phase of mania or hypomania does not fully subside or does not attain its full intensity, making the child remain overactive, impulsive, and mischievous, mimicking ADHD, conduct disorder, or related disruptive behavior disorders.[2] In general, however, children who initially develop the classical form of bipolar disorder as the predominant presentation of their illness, continue to exhibit such features whenever their illness worsens, and the children who initially manifest features of the atypical forms of the illness continue to exhibit such atypical features as the main manifestations of the illness for years to come—if not as a life-long pattern. Very likely, it is the children who start exhibiting such atypical patterns of the illness during their childhood and who are misdiagnosed as suffering from ADHD and conduct disorders, etc., who are being increasingly recognized in their adult years, by psychiatrists well versed in the varied manifestations of bipolar disorders in adults, as suffering from various forms of bipolar spectrum disorders.[1]

Children, who in later life develop the classical form of bipolar disorder (the one with discrete episodes of mania and depression and with periods of good remission or normality in between), often go through most of their childhood reasonably uneventfully, and are often, even considered model children. As mentioned before, when classical bipolar disorder presents itself in childhood, the features are very much similar to what one observes in the adult form of the illness, with allowances made for the manifestations to be slightly modified by the child's age and developmental level. Any mental health professional, with enough awareness and experience with bipolar disorder, should be able to identify the illness without much difficulty. However, in reality, children could go through many episodes of even, classical mania, without the problem being recognized for what it is, mainly because, most clinicians are not well aware of the occurrence and manifestations of this illness in children. It is indeed pathetic to see children who have been in treatment for years in major academic and research centers for ADHD, showing up with full-blown mania while their treatment with stimulants continue.

However, most of the misdiagnosis occurs with the most common presentation of bipolar disorder in childhood—the atypical form(s). It is this form of the illness that we are primarily concerned with in this chapter. Bipolar disorder of this nature presents in children, usually, with a combination of signs and symptoms described below.

It is important to keep in mind that any symptom or feature, by itself, does not indicate the presence of this illness. It is the combination of several of the features described below, occurring in clusters, in a waxing-and-waning manner, that should alert the clinician that the child may be suffering from bipolar disorder. Because of the mixed nature of their symptomatology and several problems described below intermingling in the same child, there is an overlap between several of the categories described below. My hope is to present the prominent features one usually come across in an atypical bipolar child.

Manifestations of Atypical Bipolar Disorders in Children
Difficult Temperament

Long-standing temperamental problems–often since infancy–are extremely common in children who suffer from the atypical form(s) of bipolar disorder. Parents describe these children as having been highly temperamental, generally overactive, impulsive, and difficult to deal with. They are described as having been poor sleepers during the night–often children who couldn't or wouldn't take a nap during the day when they were toddlers and preschoolers. They are demanding and explosive, given to severe tantrums that could go on for hours. Such tantrums are often triggered by their demand for one thing or another and not being satisfied with any reasonable offers or suggestions parents make. When these children throw temper tantrums, several adults may have to hold them down to prevent them from causing serious damage to themselves, others, and the environment they are in. Parents often make statements such as, "He doesn't take no for an answer," "You don't know what will set him off," "He never listened," "It's like walking on eggshells when he is around," etc. Parents often state that these children can be very "sweet" at times—but such behavior does not last long. They quickly revert to being easily angered, seemingly insensitive and impossible to deal with. According to parents and teachers, these children are highly variable in their behavior, day-to-day or time-to-time. One often hears terms such as "angel or devil," "Dr. Jekyll and Mr. Hyde," and similar descriptions when adults try to describe the behavior and functioning of these children. Parents often say that these children have a "split personality," (a term they have heard from the media and other sources dealing with psychiatric issues). What they really mean by this term is that the children are highly variable and unpredictable in their behavior, appearing normal or not too difficult to deal with, some times or days, and totally out of control and impossible to understand or deal with at other times or days. As the children enter school, their difficult to deal with temperament and behavior become obvious to teachers and other school authorities. Parents are called into the school, time and again, with complaints about their children's aggressive and unruly behavior. Many mothers state that they could never go to work or work peacefully because of the frequent calls and complaints from schools, and having to leave their place of work to go and get the children from schools at the middle of the day because of their temperamental and unmanageable behavior in school. It is not unusual to see mothers loosing their jobs time and again, as employers object to such disruptions caused by the children's school problems. Many children are recommended in-school counseling, then counseling in facilities in the community as the first effort is found insufficient, eventually many are treated with stimulant medications, placed in special educational classes or special schools, etc. In-spite of such efforts, by and large, the problems of these children would continue unabated or worsen as the years go by.

Intense Anger and Aggressive Behavior

The frequent, if not the most frequent complaint that brings bipolar children for psychiatric evaluation and treatment is their tendency to become extremely angry and engage in aggressive behavior. It is their angry and aggressive behavior in school, which does not respond to usual disciplinary measures, that more often than not, results in the school authorities insisting that the children receive psychiatric evaluation and intervention. Teachers complain that these children become extremely angry and aggressive for the slightest reason or no reason at all. They fight viciously and hurt other children and even adults. They can go through periods when their behavior is reasonable, only to enter a phase their irritability, anger, and aggression again tax the patience of everyone and complaints from other students, their parents, and teachers reach a crescendo. Their parents are at their wits end by this time.

A ten-year-old boy was brought in for psychiatric evaluation. Mother stated that he needed the evaluation so that the report could be given to a residential treatment facility where he was being considered for admission. She felt all the treatment he had received from out patient, inpatient (a major teaching hospital) and day treatment program, produced little benefit and she could not manage him at home. He had just been treated and referred from the teaching hospital mentioned before with a diagnosis of ADHD and Oppositional Defiant Disorder and had been prescribed 54 mg. of methylphenidate per day.

When seen for the evaluation, a summary of mothers complaints about his problems read: "He is too hyper…he has outbursts of anger…things are getting worse…he is breaking out (out of control aggression and behavior)…she can't handle him…he has school problems, fighting…they can't handle him…he sets fires…he breaks things…he is out of control…he goes on the subway for hours (leaves home or school without permission and rides the subway going here and there in the city for hours)…he has shop-lifted, he lies and steals…he has been picked up by the police (several times)…mother feels very angry, overwhelmed (by his problems)…"

This child had been seen in the Emergency Room of the teaching hospital, where he had most of his treatment, several times in the recent past. During the most recent visit he told the doctors there, his main problem was "I can't control my anger," and mother had stated "He wants what he wants" and that he was very angry and she could not deal with him anymore. She wanted him hospitalized. However she was advised to take him home, continue giving him methylphenidate and seek follow up treatment in an out patient clinic. He had a strong family history indicative of bipolar disorder.

This child's brief case history is indicative of severe tendency for anger, anger control problems, and aggression being major components of atypical bipolar disorder, with other features of the disorder also becoming evident as more information becomes available. It also shows how professionals have difficulty considering diagnoses other than ADHD and oppositional defiant disorder, and pharmacological treatment other than the already failed attempts at treatment with stimulants, when confronted by such problems. The plethora of problems exhibited by this child cannot be explained by ADHD or oppositional defiant disorder.

The tendency for intense anger and aggressive tendencies worsen as years go by. The damage children can inflict on others also become more problematic with advancing age. Atypical bipolar children who experience severe anger make up a large proportion of the children who engage in violent behavior. Often, adults find it difficult to understand why some children commit atrocious deeds. What we fail to understand is that, bipolar disorder induced anger is extremely intense and irrational—to the point of being "psychotic" in nature. One does not have to be delusional, or experiencing hallucinations, or a very bad person to behave in such manner. The intense emotionality of bipolar disorder and how it makes one feel and think are the driving forces behind many violent acts children and adults commit. Many children who experience intense anger and engage in severe aggressive behavior, however, may also experience command hallucinations or similar experiences, which intensify their aggressive behavior–a problem that is discussed in more detail later.

Irritability, Explosiveness, Labile mood

The difficult temperament most of these children have had, often take on intense characteristics such as their being highly irritable, explosive, combative, and behaviorally out of control. Their mood is often labile. They may become angry, excited, sad, tearful, wailing aloud etc.–all within a short period of time, which give the impression that they suffer from unusually intense emotionality and reactivity. Bipolar children (and adults), when going through a worsening of their illness (other than the depressive phase), often exhibit such emotional liability. Children, who are in such states of acute worsening of their illness, tolerate frustrations very poorly and often become verbally and physically explosive, when adults try to correct them or intervene in their problem behavior. Along with the emotional and behavioral turmoil they exhibit, they are also irrationally demanding–more so than they usually are—during such periods. Such a mixture of emotional and behavioral phenomena often prevents clinicians from recognizing the bipolar underpinnings of their turmoil.

Such children's angry, explosive behavior do not respond to the usual disciplining measures used by adults—such as sending them to their rooms, withholding privileges, suspending them from school, etc. (Such measures often make these children behave in a more violent and destructive manner.) Often, they and their parents come to the attention of child protective agencies because of the problematic parent-child interactions such situations create. Many of these children's records reveal that they may have experienced physical abuse from their caregivers. Often, professionals, who deal with these children later, assume, that their problems are entirely a direct result of the reported abuse. But the actual cause or causes are almost always more complex, such as the difficult temperamental characteristics of the children playing a provocative role, which interact with similar characteristics in the care givers, producing an unhealthy if not dangerous situation. It is extremely unusual for a child to become and remain hyperactive, impulsive, explosive, violent, etc. on a continuing basis, year after year, only because of one or a few alleged or real, past episodes of abuse. However, many professionals maintain such beliefs, based on their misunderstanding (originating in psychoanalytic and related theories) that psychopathology in children is always due to past emotional trauma. They subsequently channel all their efforts in that direction only, when dealing with these children. In the process they fail to recognize the bipolar disorder the child suffers from and which has played and continues to play a central role in the child's turbulent existence.

A great deal of misunderstanding and emotional turmoil for all concerned could be avoided, if clinicians, other professionals who deal with children—especially child abuse investigators and child welfare workers-, become knowledgeable of the subject of bipolar disorder in children. At present, most workers involved in such activities have little awareness of it. Journalists reporting "stories" on tragic incidents involving children, that indicate, that the children concerned very likely suffered from bipolar disorder and that the illness may have played a crucial role in the unfortunate incident, almost always appear to be completely oblivious of the concept of bipolar disorder in children. This is partly because of the fact that even the experts they consult and quote from in writing these "stories," also, more often than not, fail to see the obvious features of bipolar disorder in the children's histories and turmoils. This is another example of how even the most educated members of our society who deal with children's problems remain totally oblivious of the issue of bipolar disorder in children.

Intense Emotionality

Atypical bipolar children exhibit an abnormal intensity in all the emotions they experience–not just anger, though anger is often the most problematic feature. Such intense emotionality gives an unreasonable and irrational quality to these children and their actions. Such emotionality is behind the explosive and aggressive behavior that brings many of these children to clinical attention. Unfortunately, most clinicians fail to see the bipolar underpinnings in these children and consider them to suffer from ADHD, oppositional defiant disorder, conduct disorder, depressive disorder NOS, etc., only. Such failure to identify bipolar disorder, often result in the children having a very troubled and misunderstood life, with many—if not the majority–growing up into a life of intense suffering, chaos, and criminal behavior without the true nature of their problem ever being recognized. It is no wonder that, today there are more mentally ill people in the prisons of many cities than in their psychiatric hospitals.

Very Poor Frustration Tolerance

Extremely poor frustration tolerance is very often a characteristic of many of these bipolar children. Parents often say that the children have always had that problem. Whatever they want, they have to have immediately or they will have the worst, destructive tantrum. They become verbally and physically explosive, if their wishes for pleasurable objects or activities are not satisfied immediately and without question. It is not uncommon to come across a ten-year-old boy trashing the whole house, breaking windows, etc., because the parents would not immediately get him some toy or similar object he demanded. It is not unusual for parents to call for police help to control the child in such situations. Though behavior of similar nature may occur at times in children who do not suffer from bipolar disorder, what distinguish the bipolar children is the extreme intensity, frequency, and the irrational–almost bizarre–nature of such behavior. Parents find dealing with such children and their behavior an impossible and hopeless task. The children appear to loose all controls and rationality, completely taken over by the intensity of their desires. In my opinion, it is the pathological emotional intensity of these desires–an intensity that is caused by the chemistry of bipolar disorders–that makes it difficult, if not impossible, for these children to act more rationally in such situations. What, other children can let go, wait for, or modify taking the advice of parents or other concerned adults into consideration, is an impossible task for the bipolar children.

Excessively Pleasure-seeking Behavior

Children, in general, are more interested in pleasure seeking activities—a behavior they exhibit, arguably, more intensely and excessively than adults. In general, such pleasure and excitement seeking of the young are considered a normal characteristic of being young. However, children who suffer from bipolar disorder, generally exhibit an inordinately increased intensity in this behavior. They demand constant pleasure and excitement, starting, often, with an insatiable demand for toys and pleasurable activities in early childhood, graduating to demands for more and more expensive objects and freedom to do as they please. Such demanding behavior is unusual and flagrantly out of proportion to that of their peers not affected by this illness. Their unending demands for one thing after another, give them a quality of being irrational and impossible to deal with. The degree to which they crave such objects, excitement, and freedom is a continuing source of conflict between them and their parents.

Clinicians who deal with such children are often struck by how intense and irrational such demands are. Soon after one of their demands is satisfied, they come up with something else–a never-ending process that keeps the parents and caregivers perpetually frustrated. Many of these children demand immediate rewards just to come to the clinic for their appointments. They often walk into the clinic with such demands and arguments with their parent or parents, so that their whole visit, time and again, is spend on negotiating with them and appeasing them about their unreasonable and never ending demands. They throw tantrums and go into explosive and destructive rage outbursts, anywhere and everywhere, when their seemingly irrational demands are not given into immediately. As they grow older, they, often start stealing to obtain whatever they want. This often results in the clinicians giving them diagnoses such as kleptomania and conduct disorder (but the bipolar disorder that triggers such behavior almost always goes undetected). They lack the capacity to work toward obtaining pleasurable objects and activities as rewards for acceptable behavior or positive accomplishments, in any reasonable manner, frustrating their parents, and clinicians who counsel them or try to set up behavior modification programs to address such problems.

Hyperactivity and Related Problems

Very often the children who are affected by atypical bipolar disorder are hyperactive and impulsive, and so, receive a diagnosis of attention deficit hyperactivity disorder (ADHD). Many of the children may have received or may be receiving treatment with stimulant medications. **However, their hyperactivity and impulsivity are usually, highly variable from time to time. Clinicians seldom notice this fact or understand what it may mean, when they notice it.**

These children could go through days or even weeks when they are not hyperactive, but adults–including mental health professionals and psychiatrists—do not recognize or notice the significance of these quiescent periods. "It depends on what mood he is in when he wakes up in the morning," or "He has good days and bad days," are common statements parents' make. Apart from being hyperactive, most of these children are highly excitable, always trying to get involved in something that is exciting for them and in the process running into conflicts with others, time and again. Compared to their behavioral and emotional problems, especially tendency to be impulsive, explosive, and aggressive, problems of in-attention are less troublesome. Few if any of these children come to the psychiatrist because of attention problems being the main complaint. **Their attention problems appear to be secondary to their excited, action seeking, and disruptive way of life. In this sense their problems differ from the problems that are considered primary to the concept of ADHD as held presently, in which, problems of attention are considered the central and primary problem** (though this is an arguable concept with not much evidence to support it).

As in most children, the activity level and capacity to concentrate on school work often improve in many bipolar children also, temporarily, when they are given stimulant medications such as Ritalin, but sooner or later the hyperactivity and behavioral problems go through periods of worsening even though they are taking the same amount of stimulant medicines as before. Parents often say that, these children appear to be perhaps a little better when they are taking medicines such as Ritalin, but "He has his days" (when the problems get worse). During such worsening, teachers often complain that the medicine (Ritalin, Dexedrine etc.) is not working any more. They often request or demand an increase in dosage (which usually will not help and may even worsen the behavior). During such episodes, the children appear to be going through short-lived manic or hypomanic episodes (albeit, often with mixed features of excitement and labile mood). They are more hyperactive, irritable, excitable, angry, labile, and explosive—both verbally and behaviorally during such periods. It is not at all unusual to see children go through repeated episodes of such worsening, with one crisis after another caused by their out of control behavior, leading to suspensions from school, emergency room visits, attempts at hospitalizations, etc., as adults involved with them—including psychiatrists and other professionals—stay baffled or inept in figuring out what is happening. During such periods, typically, each person or group involved with the child pass the problem on to the other person or group under one pretext or another, with little beneficial effect ensuing. Professionals involved in the care of such children often blame or urge each other to take more drastic actions, such as increasing the dose of the medicines again and again, suspending the child from school, changing schools, calling for hospitalization, residential placement, etc.

In my experience, such worsening of behavior and emotional state to crisis proportions because of bipolar disorder are almost always misdiagnosed and misunderstood by emergency room doctors, if and when the children are brought there in such states. If the emergency room is busy or there is no child psychiatry in patient unit in the hospital or if it is full—as they often are in most hospitals in the urban areas-, there is an added reason for the doctors not to acknowledge the nature and seriousness of the problem. They want to avoid the predicament that if they acknowledge that the child is seriously ill, they will not be able to send the child back home with some cursory advice as usual, but rather would be "stuck" with the child in the emergency room because no one knows how to effectively deal with the problem and few admitting facilities would be interested in most of such children with their history of troublesome behavior. Usually, however, it is the inability of emergency room doctors—including psychiatrists–in identifying bipolar disorder in these children, that prevents them from getting the proper attention and consideration when they are brought there. Since these children are often very young, they will not be determined to pose an immediate "danger" to their "own life or the life of others,"–an outmoded criterion to determine if involuntary hospitalization is indicated for an adult. **Such a criterion is even more inappropriate for children in distress, whose parents are requesting voluntary hospitalization for their children. Often, doctors use such outmoded concepts to deny the children admission to the hospital.** In order to justify their refusal to provide the badly needed inpatient hospitalization for these children, doctors state and record in their cursory notes that the children are not "suicidal," or "homicidal," or "psychotic" (meaning they are not professing bizarre or dangerous delusions or acknowledging problematic hallucinations), and hence, they do not deserve inpatient treatment. **The fact that the children are totally out of control emotionally and behaviorally because of the illness and that they have become impossible to treat as out patients or be maintained at home in any reasonable manner is given little consideration.** Their families are left to cope with the problem that they have been unsuccessfully grappling with for years,—once again, and through one more crisis. In such circumstances, the child's home environment is tense and in turmoil because of the persistent, out of control, and even dangerous behavior of the child. There is no peace at home, and the family members are at their wits end. **Many incidents of child abuse occur in such situations where a parent or parents—today, often, a grand mother or even a great grand mother—is left to cope with a highly disturbed bipolar child in turmoil day after day because of the ignorance and uncaring attitude of mental health professionals responsible for admitting such children to the hospitals.**

Unlike adults who suffer from classical mania, children who are going through periods of worsening of atypical bipolar disorder may not appear to be acutely "mentally ill," to those who are unfamiliar with the illness. Rather they see such children as angry, arrogant, and "bad." Psychiatrists, other doctors, and other professionals often misunderstand that the children's problems are "behavioral only." The fact that he or she is suffering from an acute worsening of bipolar illness is seldom understood or acknowledged. So also the fact that whatever the origin, the child's behavior is out of his own control, unmanageable, and extremely distressing if not life threatening. Such children are sent home from emergency rooms time and again with a cursory suggestion for "out patient follow up." The immediate intervention the child needs for the acute bipolar disorder—usually with manic or mixed components—is neither recognized nor addressed.

Unless the supervising doctors and psychiatrists in the emergency rooms are well aware of the manifestations of bipolar disorder in children—both in its classical and atypical forms-, they cannot educate the younger doctors who are in-training and who are the primary care givers in the emergency rooms, as to, how to recognize this illness in children and how to appropriately be helpful to the children and their families.

At times the hyperactivity, impulsivity, and related phenomena in these children can reach the level of disturbance one observes in severe forms of acute mania in adults. During such acute worsening they hardly sleep and may even experience auditory hallucinations, in keeping with their heightened energy level.

A six-year-old boy was seen in his apartment by home visit because of the urgency of the situation. His mother was not able to secure an inpatient admission for him though she found his behavior extremely distressing and unmanageable at home. He had a history of being hyperactive and had a history of past treatment with stimulant medication. When seen he had been suspended from school because of extremely hyperactive, destructive, and aggressive behavior. His mother reported that during the past few weeks his behavior had abruptly worsened. He had become so hyperactive, impulsive, and restless that he seldom rested or slept. She was forced to keep him in a locked room at night, and observed how he was through a peep-hole, as he would run around and jump from furniture to furniture all night in a dangerous manner, keeping everyone in the household tense and preventing them from sleeping.

When seen he came across as pleasant and friendly but elated and excited in a pathological manner. He constantly ran and jumped over furniture, in a non-stop manner and often endangered his safety. He repeatedly climbed over furniture, tried to stand on his head on top of them and attempted to somersault repeatedly and in a dangerous manner. He was over-talkative and grandiose in his pronouncements. He admitted to hearing voices urging him to keep on doing what he was doing.

Severe Oppositional Behavior

Many of these children habitually fail to comply with the requests and directions of adults responsible for them, which bring them to the attention of school authorities as "problem children," time and again. Needless to say, parents also find such behavior extremely difficult to deal with. Clinicians often consider them as exhibiting oppositional defiant disorder.[2] These children cause enormous frustration for their parents and other adults involved with them because of such behavior. Many incidents and complaints of physical and emotional abuse of children occur in such circumstances, as the oppositional and provocative behavior of the children tax the patience of a vulnerable parent or other adults.

Refusing to do homework or having a very oppositional attitude toward homework is a prominent problem of these children from their early school years. This problem only gets worse as years go by. Many such children experience having to do even minimal homework as a frustrating, totally unjust demand placed on them. They put off doing homework, ignore it all together, lie that they do not have any homework, etc. They have an innate tendency to be irritated and distressed by any activity, such as homework, which they experience as "boring" or frustrating. Even children who are very intelligent and academically capable, exhibit such oppositional behavior that they fail one or more grades and are already in special educational programs by the time they reach junior high. It is as if they cannot stand anything other than pleasurable activities. Mothers of these children "dread" homework time.

Precocious Sexuality and Hyper-sexuality

A great many of these children exhibit precocious sexuality and hyper-sexuality. This often makes people wonder whether these children have been sexually abused, or inappropriately exposed to sexual behavior or material by their caregivers. **More often than not, this problem of precocious sexuality and hyper-sexuality occurs as an innate propensity of**

these children, similar to the hyper-sexuality seen in manic and hypo-manic adults. Such behavior appears to be primarily produced by the abnormal neurochemistry and related changes that cause bipolar disorder. Their precocious sexuality and hypersexual interests and behavior bring them into conflict with parents and other adults in authority. Such behavior also tends to produce serious complications in their lives and the lives of others, as they become older. A crucial point to remember in this connection is that, bipolar disorder has an intrinsic tendency to produce heightened sexual interests at a very young age. Any time one is dealing with a child who is exhibiting problematic precocious sexual preoccupations or behavior, bipolar disorder should be included in the differential diagnosis. This is not to say that the children's environment may not be playing a primary or contributory role in some cases.

The fact, that a child's sexual interests could be aroused precociously because of bipolar disorder, is an unknown concept to many mental health professionals. Such lack of awareness often produces unfortunate consequences, with investigators often accusing the parents or others, falsely, of causing the child's precocious or unusual sexual preoccupations and interests.

Over-talkativeness

More often than not, bipolar children are over talkative. Such over-talkativeness may happen more-or-less on a continuing basis, or in an episodic and waxing and waning manner. Severe over-talkativeness, pressured speech, and pathological elation are signs of classical mania and hypomania. However, over-talkativeness and pressured speech are not as common in children who suffer from the atypical forms of bipolar disorder, compared to their occurrence in classical mania or hypomania. Children who exhibit over-talkativeness as a prominent feature, generally are found to be suffering from the classical form of bipolar disorder: either bipolar I, or bipolar II [2]. However, their spells of elation and over talkativeness, remain, more or less, as a continuous phenomena, with only brief periods of remission, or interspersed with mild depressive episodes, when they appear under active and verbally under-productive. Along with their long lasting or continuously elated and over-talkative periods, they exhibit impatience, irritability, over-activity, impulsivity, and related phenomena though, in general, they are less angry and aggressive than the children who suffer from the atypical forms of bipolar disorder wherein elation and over-talkativeness may not be as predominant a feature. Children who suffer from the atypical forms of bipolar disorder, in comparison to those with classical forms of the illness, are less over-talkative and exhibit the pattern of irritability, intense anger, and aggression more, compared to the tendency to be elated.

In my experience, **the bipolar youngsters who are generally elated and over talkative–and thus, are more likely to be affected by the classical forms of bipolar disorder–, are less prone to violence than those who predominantly exhibit features of atypical bipolar disorder: irritability, intense anger, explosiveness, aggression, conduct problems, etc.**

Preoccupation with Ideas and Questions that are Unusual for Children of Their Age

Some of the bipolar children show unusual interest—to the point of being obsessed—and insight into the human predicament and related issues. They often obsessively ask questions about philosophical concerns, such as the meaning of life, why the world is the way it is, the concept of God, etc., in a manner that is unusual for children of their age and difficult for adults to explain to the children's satisfaction. The obsessive, persistent quality to their questioning and their inability to be satisfied with any explanations adults give them about these matters, make them appear very intelligent but at the same time as extremely unusual.

Sleep Problems

Often, parents report that these children always slept poorly. **The children often do not complain about their poor sleep—rather the problem** is their inability or lack of desire to sleep at regular hours and the annoyance and disruption it causes to other family members. They want to keep awake and remain active or playing, late into the night (in a manner that is unusual for children of their age), disturbing others, showing little concern they have school next day, ignoring the parents' pleadings, going into explosive outbursts, temper tantrums, etc., in the process. The children often state, that they are not tired and would continue to keep playing or entertaining themselves in a boisterous manner to such an extent, that bedtime is always severely conflict ridden.

Many children who are not affected by any significant emotional problems or illness, would also, often, want to postpone going to bed so that they could continue playing or watching T.V. for "some more time." However, with the bipolar children, the problem is severe and persistent to a highly problematic degree, in-spite of parents' efforts to help them establish reasonable sleep hours. Such children often say that they can do without much sleep. Children of this nature, when seen during their teens or adult life often remark "I never slept...I've always been like that." An eleven-year-old boy told me, *"I am built different,...I mean I am not like those others,...I don't have to sleep much,...I have to sleep only three hours, but I am not tired in the morning."* Parents often state that in-spite of these children often going to bed late they wake up early in the morning (though this is not always the case, as many bipolar children refuse to get up in the morning to get ready for school, setting up a conflict ridden and stressful situation for the parents from the beginning of the day itself). In contrast to this, there are times when they are reported to be sleeping excessively (most likely when they are in a depressive phase of the illness), though such reports are less frequent compared to that of their refusal or inability to sleep for sufficient hours and at proper times.

Depression

Though classical bipolar disorder with episodes of mania or hypomania is not the most common presentation of bipolar disorders in children, episodes of identifiable depression, do occur periodically in most bipolar children–even the ones who suffer from the atypical forms of it. Children, who more or less continuously exhibit hyperactivity, impulsivity, or conduct problems, become more subdued during such periods. To many uninitiated observers, these children's behavior may even appear to have improved during such periods. But on closer scrutiny, they may be found to be experiencing lack of energy, a tendency to stay home bound-compared to their usual tendency to be out seeking pleasurable activities-, an increase in vague somatic symptoms often pertaining to the head and abdomen[22,23] (the abdominal symptoms are often diagnosed as irritable bowel syndrome by physicians), and at times guilt feelings about their previous transgressions. Clinicians who evaluate children during such periods often perceive an element of depression and give them a diagnosis of depression of one type or another, but most often do not detect that the depression is part of bipolar disorder. During such periods when the depressive symptoms predominate, some children may reveal suicidal thoughts, but serious suicide attempts are fortunately rare in this younger group of children.

Usually the depressive phase of bipolar disorder, in children who suffer from the atypical forms of the illness, do not occur in clear cut long lasting episodes, but instead, appear intertwined with conduct problems and impulsivity. Such depressive episodes often do not fit neatly into the characterization of major depression in DSM IV.[2] Whether they qualify for a diagnosis of major depression as per DSM IV or not, any depressive phenomena–even short lived ones—associated with bipolar disorder have to be taken seriously, as children not only suffer because of depression, but also could become irrational and hopeless in their thinking during such periods. The risk of acting on such irrational and pessimistic thoughts generally increases with the age of the child.

It is to be kept in mind that **depressed mood is not always a prominent feature of all children who go through the depressive phase of atypical bipolar disorder. Rather what is more evident is a shift in the energy level, with the children becoming less active, less talkative, and mildly** withdrawn, compared to their usual state of being excited, overactive, talkative, boisterous, and aggressive.

Auditory Hallucinations

When auditory hallucinations occur in clear consciousness in children, first and foremost one has to consider bipolar disorder as the possible underlying problem.[24] The conventional belief is that auditory hallucinations in children occur most often due to schizophrenia. However, by and large, the more one studies the issue of auditory hallucinations in children the more one is impressed by the fact that bipolar disorder is the usual underlying problem. Often the hallucinations occur when the child is predominantly in the depressive phase. The hallucinations in such circumstances may be derogatory, or of a command nature urging the child to engage in a self destructive or self-abusive behavior. At times they may occur as voices accusing the child of past transgressions in a guilt-producing manner. When the child is not in a predominantly depressive state, he or she may experience the voices as two sides of his mind arguing, taking on the persona of good and evil, or devil and angel, etc., placing him or her in a predicament of not knowing what to do. Bipolar children, who engage in behavior such as shop lifting in a somewhat compulsive manner, often report that they experience a voice or closely related phenomena urging them to steal the object that has caught their attention. Children who frequently get into physical altercations in schools, often reveal command hallucinations or a phenomena closely resembling it urging them to fight—a reason, along with their high emotionality and intense anger, that may explain why they fight in a totally out of control and vicious manner. Teachers in special educational settings are very familiar with such children for the ferociousness and frequency of their fights and other aggressive acts, and how at times, even several adults acting together have difficulty separating or subduing such children when they start fighting or attacking other children. **The hallucinatory urgings seem to add a level of intensity and persistence to their angry, aggressive**

behavior. A frequent comment one hears from teachers about such a child is "When he fights he goes for the jugular."

Visual Hallucinations

It is a commonly accepted fact in psychiatry that visual hallucinations are usually a sign of delirium and related phenomena. This is indeed true in most cases. However, very few people are aware of the fact that visual hallucinations and related phenomena, at times, occur in children and adults experiencing bipolar disorder. Unlike in delirium, where such phenomena are often frightening, and may even force the sufferer to engage in dangerous behavior such as trying to jump out the window to avoid a dangerous situation, the visual hallucinatory phenomena that are reported by bipolar children have a matter-of-fact-quality to them. They often mention seeing a close relative who died some time back "just as you are sitting there," or a cartoon character or animal like creature and almost appear to take the experience for granted. Such reports often prompt clinicians to comment that the child has a "vivid imagination" or that the child experiences "hysteric phenomena," or may be "psychotic." Rarely such phenomena could be anxiety or fear producing, especially when it occurs at night. It is difficult to decide whether such phenomena occurring at night are illusory or hypnagogic experiences.

When the visual hallucinatory experiences are not anxiety producing or frightening, children, often do not report such experiences spontaneously, but may reveal them on careful probing aimed at eliciting such symptomatology. Though visual hallucinatory type of phenomena can, and do, occur in bipolar children, they are much less frequent compared to the frequency of auditory hallucinations. **The issue of visual hallucinations and related phenomena are highlighted here to remind clinicians that, when a child reports such phenomena as occurring in clear consciousness, bipolar disorder should be included in the differential diagnoses–not just schizophrenia or psychotic disorder NOS.**

Suicidal Tendencies and Threats

Bipolar children often talk of wanting to die or of suicidal urges, from a very young age (even from their pre-school years). This may at times be in response to loss of a loved one, or in response to what they perceive as a difficult life, but is often out of proportion to the circumstances they give as reasons for making them feel that way. At times there may not be any easily discernible reason. They often say, that they want to kill themselves and join a close relative, whom they knew, and who died either recently or sometime back. More often, they threaten to kill themselves, in response to minor frustrations, or the parents or other adults reprimanding them for their misbehavior or faults. When one hears of a child expressing death wishes or suicidal thoughts or urges–especially, repeatedly-, not only depression, but bipolar disorder also has to be considered a strong possibility. Parents often remark about such children, "He always said that." It is my experience that a majority of children referred from schools to the emergency rooms because of making suicidal statements suffer from bipolar disorder–especially if they have a history oh behavior problems also-, and the depressive phenomena are only one aspect of the disorder. **Most clinicians and lay people think of only depression when a child makes statements that he wants to die or that he wished he were dead, but few think of the depressive manifestations as a component of the bipolar disorder they may be suffering from.**

CHAPTER IV

BIPOLAR DISORDERS IN ADOLESCENCE

Though, many features of bipolar disorders are similar in younger children and adolescents, in general, the symptomatology intensifies during adolescence and is further colored by adolescence itself. Hence, the issue of bipolar disorders presenting in adolescence deserves special consideration.

The Perennial Question: normal adolescence or something more malignant

Most of us agree, that adolescents, in general, are more pleasure and excitement seeking than most, mature adults. Such behavior is seen as an integral part of being young and as a consequence or accompaniment of the hormonal changes and developmental spurt that characterize adolescence. When children enter adolescence with the accompanying hormonal changes, accelerated growth, expansion of mind's capacities, etc., the desire to explore and experience the world and the urge for romantic relationships take a big leap, bringing with it the joys, conflicts, and problems that accompany this unique phase of human development. This makes the passage through adolescence a difficult time for many youngsters and dealing with such adolescents a challenge for their parents. Most adolescents and their parents traverse this phase without major mishaps. However, for many adolescents, the surging desire to seek pleasure and excitement, and the taming of such desires—especially that of sexual instincts—that parents and society demand, prove to be very difficult. This may be partly because of their temperamental characteristics and the particular environment—family and social—that they are part of. The term "adolescent turmoil" has often been used to describe the emotional upheaval and behavior of such youngsters. In contemporary life, this often involves behaviors, such as the youngsters lessening interest in school and studies—with the resulting threat of school failure and danger of dropping out-, excessive involvement with peers and groups engaged in varying degrees of unhealthy activities, difficulty adhering to reasonable curfew, challenging parental authority to an unreasonable degree, tendency to start using or "experimenting" with cigarettes, alcohol, other drugs, etc. Their falling in and out of romantic relationships or insistence that they should be allowed to have a highly involved and intimate relationship with a boy or girl they had just recently met is another common problem.

These phenomena, that are considered within the range of diffi-cult-but-still-normal adolescence, make it difficult for adolescents them-selves, their parents, and other adults in authority, as well as professionals who deal with them to determine whether such behaviors, emotionality, and intensity are part of a somewhat difficult but nevertheless normal part of adolescence, or whether they portend, or, are manifestations of a more malignant problem or illness.

Differentiating Bipolar Disorder from Usual Adolescent Problems or Turmoil

No one can pretend that it is easy to definitely decide, whether, what one is observing is part of a somewhat difficult adolescence, or, whether it is part of a subtle—or not so subtle—bipolar disorder in-development. However, experienced observers well versed in child and adolescent bipolar disorder, can make the distinction, in most cases, sooner or later. If the distinction cannot be made fully, in spite of prolonged observations and efforts, it nevertheless is a good sign—something to be thankful for–, that at worst, the illness is at least not very severe. This brings us to a crucial fact that is always good to remember when dealing with the issue of bipolar disorder in adolescents. **Unless the history and observed phenomena** are clearly indicative that, what one is observing are the manifestations of bipolar disorder, this illness in adolescence–as in childhood also— would require prolonged on going observations, preferably as a part of ongoing treatment efforts, for many months, if not longer, before a diagnosis of bipolar disorder can be made with reasonable certainty. This fact has been emphasized in two of my previously published articles on the subject.[22,23] **Until, definitive biological tests to diagnose bipolar disorder become available as a result of future research, this is the only way to confirm bipolar disorder.**

In diagnosing bipolar disorder in adolescence, **one thing to keep in mind is that this illness is primarily one of intensity of emotions and high variability in energy level**–from very high to very low or in an uneven manner. **The illness varies a great deal in the manner in which it occurs—from mild to extremely severe in intensity and the emotional and behavioral dysfunction it creates.**

To start with adolescents who are affected by this illness are more intense in their emotionality, reactivity, and temperament. Whether it is excitement, anger, or sadness they experience them more intensely than others who are not affected by the illness. **Their desires have an intensity they cannot resist, their urges cannot wait, their anger is incendiary, their imaginations go way beyond and may even blur the distinction between fantasy and reality, their energy is too high or too low propelling their bodies into hyperactivity or making them listless and withdrawn, and their despair–if and when it happens, profound.** Of course, if the illness produces its extreme highs or lows, one would observe behavior that is grossly pathological and indicative of mental illness to even lay observers.

Most adolescents who pose such diagnostic challenges, usually would have been experiencing and exhibiting features that are problematic enough to make parents or school authorities detect the need for some form of professional evaluation and intervention. A mother of an adolescent in such a predicament, after describing some of the incorrigible behavior the adolescent had been exhibiting, pleaded in a distressed manner: "Doctor, please tell me, tell me, it is not some form of sickness." Parents, who are reasonably "normal" and who have gone through life's usual—and not very usual–trials and turmoil start getting a gnawing feeling that their youngster's unreasonable demands and out of control behavior are way beyond what they know and feel to be variations of adolescent normality. It is the psychiatrist's difficult duty, however, to tease out bipolar disorder when the evidence is convincing and to help the parents, child, and others who should be aware of the problem, come to terms with it as best as they can. This is one of the most challenging predicaments in psychiatry.

Helpful Points in Identifying Bipolar Disorder in Adolescents:

Based on my experience I consider that bipolar disorders in adolescence occur in four general forms or clusters of symptomatology.

The most common of these, primarily exhibits as an extreme exaggeration of all the emotional and behavioral problems one usually associates with a problematic adolescence. For the sake of description we will call this the atypical bipolar disorder of adolescence (similar to the atypical form of the illness described in childhood). Remember though, that **this atypical form of the illness is the most common form bipolar disorders in adolescents. It is designated as atypical, only because it differs from the conventional picture one has of bipolar disorder—the classical variety-**, in which cycles of elation and depression occur in rather easily identifiable, discrete episodes. This atypical form of the illness needs the greatest consideration in adolescents because, it is not only the most frequent form of the illness in this age group, but at the same time, the most unrecognized and misunderstood form of it also. Because of this, this atypical form of bipolar disorder in adolescence will be discussed in greater detail later, after briefly describing the four general patterns in which the illness usually manifests during adolescence.

The Four Most Frequent Manifestations of Bipolar Disorders in Adolescence

I. The Atypical Form of Bipolar Disorder

Adolescents who suffer from the atypical form of bipolar disorder have a very difficult temperament and are unstable emotionally. They are excessively and impulsively pleasure seeking, easily angered to a severe degree, and have great difficulty controlling their anger. They are prone to commit acts of violence and challenge and defy adult authority to a highly problematic degree. They generally experience significant academic and discipline problems in school, in spite of their often, impressive intellectual capacities. They tend to be unreasonably explosive in their behavior when facing frustrations or when their demands are not given into. A frequent characteristic that distinguishes them from other adolescents, who also may be somewhat problematic temperamentally is that, the temperamental and explosive behavior of adolescents who suffer from bipolar disorder are extremely severe and make them stand out as extremely difficult to deal with, compared to their peers. They also tend to make suicidal threats or gestures, repeatedly. Unlike adolescents who exhibit problem behavior or conduct disorder only, these atypical bipolar youngsters often have a history of sleep problems that usually start manifesting from a younger age–probably an indication that their physiological functioning is not harmonious and deviate from normality. Generally, they tend to keep awake till very late into the night and have difficulty getting up in the morning and attending school. Parents and others, who deal with them, find them to be very difficult, if not impossible deal with, and incorrigible. They often engage in physically aggressive and violent behavior toward others, which may bring them to the attention of school authorities and law enforcement officials repeatedly. They are highly crisis prone, going from one problem situation to another, severely taxing the capacities and resources of people who deal with them. They are prone to abuse alcohol and drugs from a young age. They are prone to depression, which may be transient, subtle, and atypical in its own manifestation also.

This atypical form of bipolar disorder however is not unique to adolescence. Many adults also suffer from this form of the illness, which may have surfaced during childhood or adolescence, but may have gone unrecognized, often being misunderstood as a personality disorder. Many of them become entangled in a life of chaos and criminal behavior.

The behavior patterns and symptomatology exhibited and experienced by adolescents who suffer from the atypical form of bipolar disorder, will be described in greater detail later.

II. Bipolar Disorder with Persistent Hypomanic Features

The second, common pattern of bipolar disorder in adolescence is one in which hypomanic features persist almost as a baseline phenomenon, with no consistent or long lasting period of normal (euthymic) mood. The baseline hypomanic state is similar to the bipolar II hypomania[2], except that the hypomanic state is persistent and is essentially the predominant or baseline mood and behavior state of the affected adolescent. Such a phenomenon may not be unique to adolescents, as many adults also experience and exhibit this form of bipolar disorder, though it has not been studied and written about as extensively as the classical forms of bipolar disorder.

In the hypomanic state features of elation do not reach the height and intensity of a full-blown manic episode. Those who experience hypomania are, however, abnormally elated, euphoric, overactive, and over-talkative. They generally sleep less or need less sleep than the average person. Their judgment may be compromised at times because of their tendency to be excitable, excessively pleasure seeking, and somewhat impulsive. They experience brief episodes of depression or dysphoria, during which their energy level and activity are decreased and they may sleep excessively.

Since adolescents are generally energetic and pleasure seeking, there is a greater chance, that this form of the illness, when it occurs in them, may not be recognized for what it is, even when it is producing considerable disruption in their lives. Though, at times defying and challenging of adult authority and prone to excessive pleasure seeking, being somewhat impulsive, etc., these youngsters, in general, are not as aggressive, violence prone, or difficult to deal with as youngsters who suffer from the atypical form of bipolar disorder mentioned before. For one thing, adolescents who exhibit this persistent hypomanic pattern are euphoric, gregarious, and friendly in general, which may preclude the tendency for severe, defiant, and aggressive behavior to a degree. However, youngsters in this group may experience transient delusions or hallucinations, either when they are in the hypomanic state, or in the depressive state (perhaps more often when they are in the depressive state). In general, they tend to be more cooperative with treatment than the youngsters in the atypical bipolar group. The problems of excessive pleasure seeking, impulsivity, or episodes of depression are the reasons, which bring most of these youngsters into psychiatric treatment.

III. Classical Bipolar Disorder (Bipolar I)

The third common type of presentation of bipolar disorder in adolescence is the classical form of the illness–bipolar disorder I.[2] This form of the illness was originally referred to as manic-depressive illness or manic-depressive psychosis, because of the discrete episodes of mania or depression with or without hallucinations and delusions, which characterized the illness. Often, this form of the illness ushers in as a severe depression during adolescence, with or without mood congruent hallucinations and delusions, usually precipitated by an upsetting event. This type of presentation of the illness with depression and "psychosis," is often mistaken for schizophrenia. Later on, the bipolar nature of the illness is revealed, when episodes of classical mania with pathological elation, hyperactivity, over talkativeness, and grandiosity emerge in an unmistakable form.

IV. Persistent or Recurrent Depression with Brief Spells of Hypomania

The fourth type of presentation of bipolar disorder in adolescence—perhaps the least common but nevertheless highly problematic and causing diagnostic confusion when it occurs-, is that of persistent or recurrent depression and withdrawal as the main characteristics, with rare episodes of usually short lived spells of mild elation and over activity of a mild hypomanic nature.

During the episodes of depression and severe withdrawal, the youngsters are not able to function in any reasonable manner, and usually remain homebound, even, neglecting self-care. The main difficulty in dealing with this type of problem is that, the long episodes of depressive withdrawal often do not respond to commonly used antidepressants easily, and the response is often incomplete when it occurs or overshoots to hypomania, only to revert back into the state of withdrawal again. Because of their persistent withdrawal and inability to participate in life in any effective manner, these youngsters are almost always misdiagnosed as suffering from schizophrenia and treated with neuroleptics, which may even worsen their condition. These adolescents, unless their condition is properly diagnosed and effectively treated, drop out of school and become totally homebound, even bed ridden most of the time. They are often troubled by suicidal thoughts. Professionals and agencies involved in their care have to have great deal of understanding of the nature of these youngsters problems and commitment to their treatment—including capacity for outreach efforts-, to successfully undertake the treatment of these youngsters and to reverse the process of extreme withdrawal and depression, which could even become life threatening.

One important fact to remember about this type of bipolar depression is that the depressive phase can be very prolonged. Often people think of depression as something that lasts for a few months at best, followed by recovery or switch to manic or hypomanic phase. But, in this type of bipolar depression, the depressive phase can last for the better part of a year followed by partial recovery or brief period of hypomania and then reversal into another prolonged period of depressive withdrawal. Many clinicians, often notice the state of withdrawal only, and consider it a manifestation of schizophrenia.

Many of these youngsters need a period of hospitalization to successfully treat their condition, but since they may not appear severely depressed, when seen briefly in a clinic or emergency room visit, the seriousness of the condition is often not recognized. Many such youngsters end up living a life of chronic incapacitation. Suicide is an ever-present danger in many such youngsters.

Describing the various forms in which bipolar disorders occurs in adolescents is not a very easy task. Any description of complex and variable behavior patterns and symptomatology of this nature has inherent limitations. More over, the patterns described above are not always mutually exclusive. For example, adolescents described in any of the above categories can have episodes of classical mania, hypomania, depression, mixed phases, episodes of dysphoric mania (where the predominant mood is dysphoric but the behavior is more akin to mania), etc.[11,12] with or without hallucinations or delusions at any time in their lives.

As mentioned before, atypical bipolar disorder, described briefly before, in my opinion, is the most common but most misunderstood and misdiagnosed form of this illness in adolescence. Understanding the manifestations of this form of the illness, is the single most important skill psychiatrists and other clinicians can acquire, to improve the plight of countless number of these youngsters who presently go misunderstood, misdiagnosed, and improperly treated. It is rare, if not impossible, to find detailed description of its manifestations in the published literature dealing with children and adolescents. Since making people aware of the nature and manifestations of this form of the bipolar disorder is the main purpose of this book, a detailed description of it is given below along with discussion of relevant issues.

The Most Frequent but Most Misunderstood: Atypical bipolar disorder

Atypical bipolar disorder in adolescents usually manifests with the following features:

Difficult Temperament

Parents and others who have known the adolescents who suffer from the atypical form of bipolar disorder report that these youngsters have had a difficult temperament since early childhood. They have a history of having been highly irritable, demanding, difficult to console or satisfy, and given to severe temper tantrums from a very young age. Instead of such temperamental characteristics becoming subdued with time, as they do in most children, in this group of children, they continue to persist or worsen. During adolescence, their explosive temper, very low frustration tolerance, excessive and irrational demands, etc., form a volatile mixture, making it extremely difficult for parents, school authorities, and others to deal with them. It is such complaints and problems that bring most of these adolescents for psychiatric evaluation and treatment.

Intense Anger

Tendency to be easily angered to a pathological degree, and inability to control their aggressive behavior when angry, are frequent characteristics of these adolescents. The intensity and out of control nature of their anger, however, is often not understood for its bipolar origins–one of the main reasons why this disorder goes unrecognized for years, if not the whole life time. Adults responsible for these youngsters, usually consider them to be having an "anger control problem," which they solely attribute to their being "bad" or to their poor upbringing. These youngsters have a history of having had a "bad temper" which has steadily gotten worse, in spite of parents' and professionals' attempt to correct their behavior. They are often described as having a "foul-mouth", as they use extremely profane language, when angry. Parents often make statements, such as, "You should hear his language…the cursing…I don't know where he learns it from, nobody in the house talks that way." They storm out of the classroom if the teachers place the slightest demands on them or reprimand them, even mildly, for one reason or another. These youngsters often get into physical fights in school, threaten, and even assault their teachers. School authorities often find these youngsters uncontrollable and a threat to the safety of others. They are often suspended or dismissed from school after school because of their incorrigible behavior and aggression. They generally end up receiving little meaningful education.

Excessively Pleasure-seeking Behavior

Excessively pleasure-seeking behavior, described previously in bipolar children, continue as a problem into adolescence, except that it becomes even more problematic in adolescence. Their pleasure seeking behavior now extends way beyond usual childhood desires and excitements. Their insatiable demands for money and unwise spending habits are a constant source of friction at home. Compared to other adolescents who also desire a great deal of money and excitement, the demands and spending habits of these youngsters come across as extremely unreasonable, to the point of being irrational, if not bizarre, to their parents and other adults who are good judges of adolescent behavior patterns and norms. They often seek total freedom from all parental and social constraints, such as reasonable curfew, school attendance, etc., and often stay out all night long–even days together— without parental permission. Many engage in sexual activities indiscriminately and with multiple partners, repeatedly, with all its unhealthy and dangerous ramifications. It is the persistence and intensity of such patterns of behavior that makes these youngsters stand out from other troubled adolescents who also may indulge in some such transgressions occasionally.

Overactivity

Many of these adolescents have a history of having been overactive, if not frankly hyperactive, at least at times or phases in their lives. Though, they may not be as hyperactive and impulsive as they were when they were younger, they generally continue to be very active, and exude high energy, which they often channel into problematic activities, bringing them into conflict with their parents and society. Many of them, may have been given a diagnosis of ADHD from the time they were younger. Many would have had counseling, psychotherapy, behavior modification, and treatment with stimulant medications such as Ritalin and Dexedrine, often with poor or inconsistent results. Asked about their energy level, they often identify themselves as youngsters who have a great deal of energy—a fact supported by their parents also. "I have a lot of energy," is a comment one often hears from these youngsters.

Insomnia and Other Erratic Sleep Patterns

Inability to sleep well is a persistent problem with most of these youngsters. Often, their parents state that these youngsters slept poorly all their lives—a fact that the youngsters themselves corroborate. However, only at times do these youngsters perceive this as a problem. More often, they state, that they only need a few hours of sleep and that is the way they always have been. "I could never fall asleep" or "Who wants to sleep, sleep is a waste of time," and similar comments are what one hears often from these youngsters. Most adolescents, often, would want to go to sleep only late at night, so that they could stay up talking to friends on the phone, or exchanging messages on the internet, "hang out" with friends until a late hour, watch late night television programs, etc., but with these youngsters, the sleep problem is way beyond what happens with most adolescents. They often state that they are still "revved up," "have a lot of energy," when it is bedtime for most people. They keep awake and continue to engage in pleasurable activities, causing conflict between them and their parents. Because of keeping awake until very late on weeknights, they have difficulty getting up in time for school next morning. Such behavior leads to poor attendance, poor grades, and often dropping out from high school.

Many of these youngsters exhibit, the so-called, "reversal-of-sleep" pattern or "reversal-of-day-night" pattern. In such situation, the youngsters keep awake late into the early morning hours engaged in one inappropriate activity or another and go to sleep only by the early morning hours, but stay asleep through most of the succeeding day. They usually get up from bed by only the late afternoon or evening, after which, the disturbed sleep and behavior pattern starts all over again. Whether this reversal-of-day-night pattern is an inherent problem caused by bipolar disorder, or if it is due to the change in habit, because of keeping awake late into the night and subsequently needing to sleep late into the day is often impossible to ascertain. One thing is sure, once they fall into this dysfunctional pattern, very few of the youngsters are able to establish a normal pattern of sleep or functioning. Few of such youngsters complete high school, in any reasonable manner.

Some adolescents, though going to sleep only at a late hour, state that when they wake up in the morning they feel refreshed nevertheless. Such youngsters often exhibit signs of hypomania. Their falling asleep only very late at night, but getting up energized early in the morning appear to be related to the increased energy level and decreased need for sleep that is characteristic of mania and hypomania. One such youngster told me, "I am built that way,…I mean, I am not like those other people, I don't need much sleep." These youngsters, at times say, that they want to keep awake and enjoy life, that if they go to sleep at an appropriate time, they feel, they are loosing precious time to enjoy life, or that they are loosing out because the whole world is having "a good time" when they are asleep. They can't stand the thought (irrational of course), that life is passing them by when they are asleep.

Though, many of the bipolar youngsters who experience various types of sleep problems do not complain of their inability to sleep well, some do complain at times, that their inability to fall asleep or stay asleep is an annoying problem. Unlike most youngsters who suffer from insomnia that is troublesome to them and who stay in bed unhappy about not being able to sleep, most youngsters with atypical bipolar disorder, more often than not, would not go to bed at a proper time. Rather, they stay up remaining active, engaging in various inappropriate activities, often disturbing the sleep of others in the house. It is conceivable, that their sleep difficulty is upsetting to them when they are in a predominantly depressed or dysphoric mood and not troublesome to them when they are predominantly in a more energetic state. However, since the mood and energy states of these atypical bipolar youngsters are more often intertwined or mixed, it is difficult to correlate their sleep patterns with their mood states, clearly and always. This is in contrast to the sleep problems of the youngsters suffering from classical bipolar disorder, who tend to sleep very little when they are elated and excessively when they are in the depressive phase.

Parents, often give a history of sleep problems occurring in the families of youngsters suffering from atypical bipolar disorder. The mother, of an adolescent girl who exhibited the type of sleep difficulties described above and who recently had been diagnosed as having bipolar disorder, stated, "It runs in my family, I could never sleep,…I need something for sleep,…my mother was the same way, she slept only three hours a night." This mother, herself, had been exhibiting signs of bipolar disorder similar to that of her daughter, and readily acknowledged that the daughter was ill with such a problem, but could not understand or accept the fact that she also suffered from a similar illness—a situation one comes across time and again with parents who suffer from bipolar disorder but refuses to acknowledge the fact.

Erratic Eating Patterns or Eating Disorders

Many adolescents suffering from atypical bipolar disorder are also affected by eating problems or disorders. **Since bipolar disorder, first and foremost, is very much a problem of severe emotional intensity, it is conceivable that the adolescents who suffer from it are more prone to being affected—to an obsessive degree—by the desire to be thin, as present day social values dictate.** Since such dictates of society, arguably, have a greater–even tyrannical–impact during adolescence, it is understandable that eating disorders appear commonly during that period of life. The disastrous combination of biological vulnerabilities induced by bipolar disorder and adolescence, it seems, makes the psychological impact of such social dictates about thinness and dieting take hold of these youngsters in an intense and pathological manner.

Bipolar adolescents with eating problems, mostly exhibit the anorectic pattern, though tendency for this pattern to intermingle with bulimia is also seen at times. Since, obsessive-compulsive problems are frequent in bipolar youngsters, their eating disorders often appear to be a manifestation of obsessive fears of weight gain and compulsive food avoidance to ward off such fears. **The bipolar youngsters' intense emotional sensitivity, due to the biological abnormalities of bipolar disorder, appears to underlie both the eating disorder and the obsessive fears, which accompany it.** Such emotional intensity, makes their doubts and fears more intense and difficult to ignore or deal with, compared to that of other youngsters who do not suffer from such biological vulnerabilities, and hence, are able to deal with the tyrannical social dictates in a more rational and flexible manner. However, occasionally, one also sees some atypical bipolar youngsters who have been "picky eaters" from infancy, and whose eating problems do not appear to be related to concerns about weight gain, but rather may be directly related to the biological changes that underlie bipolar illness itself. **In many of such children bipolar disorder** appears to interfere with neurochemical or physiological factors that control appetite, desire for food intake, and feelings of satiety.

Children and adults, who are experiencing a classical manic episode, often overeat, feel extremely hungry, and desire food to an excessive degree. The biological changes that accompany mania appear to increase their metabolism, resulting in these manifestations. So also, loss of appetite is a usual feature of most types of depressions. Given the drastic changes in energy fluctuation that occur in bipolar disorder, it is understandable, how a youngster experiencing bipolar disorder would also experience abnormal eating patterns, even if the social pressures to remain thin may not be a significant contributing factor. In my experience, the erratic eating patterns in many bipolar adolescents (and children) do not appear to be only a problem of societies where the desire to be thin is paramount. However, there is also little doubt, that bipolar disorder makes adolescents more vulnerable to societal dictates about thinness and attractiveness, and this in turn makes them more prone to develop eating disorders such as anorexia.

Extreme Concerns about Physical Appearance

Most people agree that adolescents, as a group, are very concerned about their physical appearance and attractiveness. The desire to beautify ones body, to be clothed in attires that would bring them appreciative attention from their peers, in short, to be admired for their looks and style, are all part and parcel of being an adolescent. Hence, experimentation in making themselves appear very attractive is a normal preoccupation of adolescents—perhaps more so than of other age groups. With youngsters who suffer from atypical bipolar disorder (and in the manic and hypomanic states of classical bipolar disorder also), this desire goes beyond the bounds of normality, to the pathological, so that their tendency to beautify their body, whether by make up, attention-getting-attire, hair style, etc., often reach the point of flamboyance. These adolescents overdo the fashions and trends of the day to such a degree that, they are often considered unusual–if not bizarre-, by even their peer group who share many of their concerns, desires, and preoccupations about physical appearance. Many of the atypical bipolar youngsters, come across as flamboyant, driven by their preoccupations about stylish clothes, hair coloring and style–changing one outrageous style to another in rapid succession-, multiple body piercing, tattooing, etc. Some times, only they seem to be oblivious of how strange and inappropriate their appearance may be. Underneath this tendency to overdo, lies the fears, insecurities, and doubts the bipolar illness creates because of the extreme over sensitivity of emotions, it causes. **In this sense, bipolar disorder can be viewed as an illness of emotional intensity and over-sensitivity of an extreme degree—whether the emotions are of joy, sadness, anger, fear, or one of obsessive, self-doubt.**

Some times, such adolescents become so concerned about their appearance that, they are unable to leave the house to go to school, unless they feel totally satisfied with every aspect of their appearance and attire. This problem is usually more pronounced in girls. They start getting panicky the night before, about how they will look, what they will wear, etc. Often, when the morning arrives they are unable to go to school, as they are dissatisfied and doubt-ridden about their appearance and attire. They frequently do not attend school because of such concerns and drop out because of the poor attendance and grades. These phenomena, at times, could approach or even satisfy the criteria given for obsessive-compulsive disorder or body dysmorphic disorder.[2] In fact many adolescents who suffer from atypical bipolar disorder meet the criteria for these disorders also. **Rather than consider them as co-morbid problems, I consider them as part and parcel of the bipolar problem itself, caused by the intense emotional sensitivity it creates, making the sufferer extremely vulnerable to cultural dictates.** This is also in keeping with the burgeoning concept of bipolar spectrum disorders, in which, such combined features intermingle frequently in people suffering from bipolar disorders.[1,6,19] Whether such mixed symptomatology is manifestation of one illness, or a combination of several discrete illnesses, is a question that could only be fully settled when biological tests to identify bipolar disorder and other psychiatric illnesses become available.

Tendency to Smoke and Use Alcohol and Drugs to a Highly Problematic Degree

Many of the adolescents suffering from the atypical form of bipolar disorder, start smoking, and drinking alcohol, from a very young age and to a highly problematic degree. Such behavior often starts even before adolescence, in many such youngsters.

The tendency to start smoking and drinking from a very early age, is another example of the inherent tendency of these youngsters, to be drawn into anything they experience as exciting. In this sense, they are also more vulnerable to unhealthy peer group influences than other youngsters who are not genetically predisposed to bipolar disorder. The emotional intensity and vulnerability caused by bipolar disorder also appear to make them vulnerable to addiction to other drugs. They often gravitate to using drugs, such as marijuana and other hallucinogens, and often end up becoming dependent on cocaine, and opioids, by early adulthood. **One comes across such histories of alcohol and drug use starting in adolescence–or even earlier-, often, when dealing with adult drug users who exhibit features of bipolar disorder and who give a history indicative of the illness surfacing in them during their childhood or adolescence, usually in its atypical forms.** Most people who suffer from bipolar disorder of the atypical variety under discussion presently and who are troubled by alcohol and drug abuse, often go through treatment in alcohol and drug treatment settings for years, without the central destabilizing factor of their life—bipolar disorder—being recognized and treated. **Adolescents, and adults suffering from bipolar disorder, rarely stay free of substance use, unless the primary contributing cause for their substance dependence–bipolar illness—is recognized and effectively treated.** Unless our drug treatment centers have the capacity to institute effective psychiatric evaluations and treatment to address illnesses such as bipolar disorder this sad state of affairs will not improve.

The alcohol and drug abuse problems of the bipolar youngsters is often much more severe and persistent than that of other youngsters not affected by this illness. Many adolescents and young adults go through periods of the so called "experimentation" with substances of abuse, but are able to overcome such tendencies, with minimal or no outside help. However, many, if not most of the bipolar youngsters who start using alcohol and drugs become dependent on them. **Whenever a substance-abusing adolescent is seen for psychiatric evaluation, bipolar disorder, especially in its atypical form, should be ruled out.**

Hyper Sexuality

A high proportion of adolescents exhibiting bipolar disorder of the type we are presently discussing, exhibit hyper sexuality, which often starts manifesting even before they enter adolescence (note the section on hyper sexuality and precocious sexuality in the childhood section). The intensification of sexual drive during adolescence, mostly brought on by hormonal and other physiological changes of adolescence, is well known. Bipolar disorder–specifically the biochemical changes that cause the manic component—intensifies these tendencies, desires, and urges to a highly problematic degree. The resulting, pathologically intensified sexual drive and preoccupations, lead to sexually impulsive and risk taking behaviors with their unfortunate consequences.

Adolescent girls, so affected, tend to expose themselves repeatedly to environments where boys and men could sexually exploit and abuse them. Adolescent boys, affected by bipolar disorder, repeatedly engage in sexual escapades and often leave the lives of many girls troubled and tarnished. Many girls suffering from bipolar illness become pregnant, even repeatedly, because of their hyper-sexuality and impulsivity. These are trying circumstances for parents. Counseling and other measures often have little impact in modifying the hypersexual and impulsive behavior of these adolescents.

Bipolar illness complicates and intensifies the usual problems of adolescence, producing an exasperating circumstance for all concerned and a disastrous adolescence for the youngster affected by it.

Often, the brief but intense romantic and sexual involvements of such adolescents and the attendant disappointments, result in violent and suicidal behavior. They, often try to prevent a partner from breaking off the relationship, by intimidation and threats of physical harm to themselves or the partner. Clinicians, evaluating adolescents in such crisis situations, often fail to recognize the bipolar disorder, which is causing the abnormal intensity and chaos in these youngsters' lives. **Many adolescents, who commit violent acts, attempt suicide, or engage in self-mutilation–even when such behavior is triggered or is in response to a life situation-, suffer from the atypical form of bipolar disorder, though this fact is seldom recognized.**

Suicide Attempts, Gestures, and Self-mutilation

With the adolescents affected by atypical bipolar disorder, one comes across frequent episodes of suicide attempts or gestures, by taking overdoses of medicines or by other means. Girls, often slash their wrists or other parts of the body, or take minor overdoses of over the counter or prescription medicines. Clinicians, who evaluate such youngsters in emergency rooms, often mistakenly consider such behavior as "only manipulative" or "attention seeking." Often, these episodes are triggered by interpersonal conflicts, disappointments, or stresses and hence, are considered only "reactive." Such youngsters, when seen in emergency room visits, are usually given a diagnosis of adjustment reaction,[2] or depressive disorder NOS and sent home, at times with a prescription for antidepressants. The fact however is that, youngsters who react most intensely to situations in these manners are often suffering from bipolar disorder. Again, **the point to keep in mind is that, bipolar disorder–because of the emotional intensity it causes–produces intense behavioral and emotional reactions to environmental stresses, in those affected by it. A "reactive** component" does not preclude the existence of bipolar disorder. On the contrary, the more intense the reaction is, greater the possibility of bipolar disorder—especially the atypical type.

Many adolescents, who are initially diagnosed as suffering from adjustment reactions, on closer scrutiny, or later on, will be found to have bipolar disorder. Just because environmental precipitants can be found, it cannot be concluded that the problem is not one of bipolar disorder. Among the "reactive" catastrophes one encounter in adolescents, a significant number are due to the intense reactivity caused by bipolar disorder, which makes such youngsters feel more intensely and "act out "more vehemently than other youngsters experiencing similar stresses. **It is the combination of bipolar disorder induced sensitivities and environmental pressures that often produce disastrous behavioral consequences in adolescence.**

In this connection it is useful to keep in mind a formula similar to the one mentioned before:

Severe behavior problems or conduct disorder or features of ADHD+suicide attempt=? Bipolar disorder

In my experience, a high proportion, if not the majority of children referred by schools for urgent evaluation because of suicidal gestures or threats, if carefully evaluated, will be found to be suffering from bipolar disorder.

"Mood Swings"

"Mood swings" is a term often used by professionals, patients, parents, and lay people. It is a term that defies easy description but does suggest a tendency for instability and abrupt variability in emotional state and behavioral patterns. In general, it is used in connection with people, whose emotional states and behavior change problematically, quickly, frequently, and in an unpredictable manner. Their mood often shifts from being happy or elated, to angry, depressed, or dysphoric, quickly and without sufficient reason. The intensity and manner in which such changes occur are out of proportion to the life circumstances of the time. Most adolescents, and others also, experience, shifting from a happy to unhappy mood and vice versa, in response to day-to-day events. But, such mood changes are not as intense or highly problematic and are perceived by most observers to be within the normal behavioral responses of a reasonable young person. What makes the mood swings or shifts of the atypical bipolar adolescents unusual, is their intensity, and how they occur for trivial reasons or no discernable reason at all. **It is a manifestation of their volatile nature itself.** Many parents say, that they feel like walking on eggshells when these adolescents are around, as they do not know what will trigger them into an explosive outburst or out of control behavior.

These mood swings are not exactly the mixed mood states or rapid shifts from mania to depression described in DSM IV[2] or bipolar literature in adults, though a complete teasing apart of such phenomena may be difficult. The so-called mixed mood states occur when features of pathological elation and depression occur at the same time or within a brief period of each other. Difficult as it may be to conceive for people unfamiliar with the vagaries of bipolar disorder, clinicians who often deal with bipolar patients, come across people who are in a troubled and unsettled state, but their presentation is neither clearly manic nor depressed. Typically their mood fits the description of being "labile," meaning highly variable and unsettled. Significant lability of mood is a very strong indicator of bipolar disorder. The terms "bipolar disorder mixed," "dysphoric mania," etc., have been used in the adult bipolar literature to describe the symptomatology of such patients. So also, the "rapid cycling" bipolar disorder[2] is more clear-cut in its presentation and easily identifiable as such. Here the sufferer goes through episodes of classical mania or hypomania which can be identified as such easily—the episodes, often lasting a day, few days, or weeks usually. These phases alternate with similarly short lasting episodes of anergic and withdrawn depressive phases, in which the person appears unusually quiet if not very withdrawn, and often sleeping excessively—even catatonic in some cases. They become manic or hypo-manic again within a short period, and the cycle repeats itself. At times the depressive phase can be an anxious or agitated one.

In contrast, the mood swings or shifts of atypical bipolar disorder are more temperamental in quality as if it is part of the very make up of the person. They do not attain the true manic or hypomanic quality, nor do they exhibit characteristics of a major depression. The mood swings or shifts of the atypical bipolar adolescent, is usually triggered by anything that they perceive as annoying, provocative, or disappointing to them, which, their peers not affected by the illness would be able to handle in a more reasonable manner. Many of these youngsters are described as "moody" by those who know them well, and as having an "anger control problem" because of their "hair-trigger" temper. Many such youngsters are referred for anger management training these days, which may be helpful to a degree, but the underlying bipolar problem goes unrecognized and continues to cause havoc.

Involvement with Weapons

Adolescents—especially boys–who suffer from atypical bipolar disorder often develop a tendency to be excessively fascinated by, and interested in possessing knives, guns, and other dangerous weapons from a very young age. They often carry these weapons, which give them a sense of power and excitement, to protect them from real or imagined enemies. They often feel threatened because they have history of being involved in con-flicts and fights, frequently, and expect retaliation. At times the weapons are intended to just intimidate others. Some of these youngsters sleep with a knife or another weapon under their pillow, as they experience an ill-defined paranoia. Clinicians note the paranoid tendencies in such young-sters but seldom recognize the underlying atypical bipolar disorder.

In toady's world, where gun violence by adolescents is increasing to an alarming degree, it is imperative, that all youngsters who have a ten-dency for aggression and involvement with weapons–especially guns-, if

they are brought to the attention of clinicians, should be evaluated specifically, for atypical bipolar disorder. There is little doubt in my mind that many such youngsters will be found to be suffering from the atypical form of bipolar disorder. Usually they have a history of long standing behavioral and emotional problems caused by bipolar disorder but misunderstood for ADHD or conduct disorder, and the like.

When clinicians hear of a history of an adolescent involved in violence with weapons, they automatically think of conduct disorder, but seldom consider the possibility of bipolar disorder. Many such misunderstood youngsters end up receiving little meaningful treatment and often end up committing serious violence later in their lives. Today our prisons hold many such teenagers and young adults, with their mental illness–most often atypical bipolar disorder—unrecognized.

Involvement in Gangs

Adolescents who suffer from the atypical form of bipolar disorder are very prone to involvement in gangs and similar groups now prevalent in our cities. **The high energy level, thrill seeking tendencies, tendency to be irrationally daring and aggressive, craving for camaraderie at any cost, poor judgment, and related tendencies of the bipolar youngsters, make them very vulnerable to involvement with gangs.** Older gang members find the bipolar youngsters' daring characteristics and penchant for aggression, attractive characteristics for their violence-ridden ventures, and exploit the youngsters to commit violent and illegal activities that others are afraid of.

Run-a-way Behavior

The tendency to run away from home or stay away from home without parental consent for prolonged periods of days or weeks, repeatedly, is often a common problem with the atypical bipolar adolescents. They may run away in response to conflicts with parents about one issue or another or may just stay away from home, seeking pleasure and thrill with their peer group or others. During such escapades they engage in unhealthy and dangerous activities of one type or another. They tend to repeat such behavior time and again, in spite of intervention by authorities—including the police and family courts-, seemingly unconcerned of the distress such behavior causes to their family members and the disruption it causes in their own lives. **Whenever evaluating an adolescent who engages in repeated run-a-way behavior, look for history and signs that point to atypical bipolar disorder.**

Years of Psychotherapy and Treatment with Stimulants, but Little Improvement

Often, apart from the presenting symptomatology and family history, what makes one suspect bipolar disorder in these adolescents is the fact that months or years of treatment efforts through various psychotherapeutic efforts, disciplinary measures, and even treatment with stimulants such as Ritalin and Dexedrine, have produced no consistent or lasting improvement in these children. **They may appear to be slightly better for short periods of time, but sooner or later their problems intensify, all over again, to crisis proportions. Such a history should alert clinicians to the strong possibility of bipolar disorder** being the central destabilizing problem of these youngsters.

Intermittent Periods of Improvement in Behavior Followed by Worsening

Adolescents who suffer from bipolar illness of the atypical variety, in general, do not experience sustained improvement, or full remission of their symptomatology for prolonged periods of time—compared to classical bipolar illness, in which, such periods of prolonged remissions usually occur. Nevertheless, even youngsters who exhibit the atypical form of the illness, frequently go through periods when their behavior and functioning are less problematic. However, these improved states do not last long.

Often, within weeks or a few months the behavioral worsening appears again for no apparent reason, pointing to the true nature of the problem: bipolar disorder. **In out patient settings, when one is involved in ongoing treatment with these youngsters, this pattern of periodic worsening of behavior and functioning should alert one to the strong possibility of bipolar disorder.** Often, the youngsters and their parents drop out of treatment once the problems appear to have subsided to a degree and come back when the problems erupt again into a crisis situation. This pattern of on–and-off involvement in treatment, is similar to how, many people engage in treatment for other chronic illnesses such as arthritis, bronchial asthma, etc.,—coming back for treatment when the problem exacerbates, but trying to put it out of mind or just live with it when the symptoms are not too troublesome. **This type of involvement in treatment is understandable, as most people do not want to disrupt their lives or become anxious about constant doctor visits if they can avoid it. People dislike reminders that they are mentally ill–that too, with an illness for which there is no cure and the medicines available often producing unpleasant side effects.** These problems are much more pronounced with adolescents who suffer from atypical bipolar illness.

To start with, few of them want to believe or admit they are ill. This may even be due to the very nature of the illness itself, which prevents the capacity to develop self-awareness. **No one wants to carry the fear and stigma of mental illness—least of all adolescents.** They dislike psychiatric treatment and taking medications to improve their behavior. Parents also would rather believe and hope that somehow or other the problem would go away. This happens, especially, since most of the manifestations of this illness are exaggerations—albeit severe, even grotesque exaggerations—of problems many adolescents experience and exhibit, at least occasionally in their lives.

Episodes of Depression or Withdrawal

Even the adolescents who exhibit, more or less, continuing excitability and behavioral problems, at times go through periods when they appear quiet, withdrawn, and even depressed in an uncharacteristic manner. Often there is no good explanation as to why this may be happening. For adults, especially school authorities, such periods are at times a welcome change, as it is much easier to deal with these youngsters when they are in such states than when they are excited and disruptive. Often, therapists and other professionals who treat such youngsters perceive it as an improvement. The youngsters may or may not perceive they are experiencing depression, or report or admit to being depressed during such periods. More often, they report they feel tired or that they don't have much energy. In this context, **it is important to remember that bipolar disorder is an illness causing unevenness in energy regulation, one in which there is often an abundance of energy propelling one to impulsive activity, and sometimes, in contrast, little energy, making one feel tired and withdrawn.** These episodes of depression or withdrawal in atypical bipolar disorder are often short lived, usually lasting only days or weeks at a time. When they do occur, they are quite discernible to someone who knows the youngster well. Any psychiatrist who may have been treating such a youngster and who is knowledgeable of the manifestations of atypical bipolar disorder in youngsters, will be able to understand what the phenomena represents. Unfortunately, in reality, more often than not, the significance of such short-lived phenomena is seldom recognized.

At times, such depressive episodes appear as classical depressions with hypersomnia, which occurs in anergic depressive states, or with troublesome insomnia. They are at times accompanied by feelings of sadness, guilt feelings (often about indiscretions when their behavior was out of control), inferiority feelings, somatic preoccupations (excessive worry about minor physical problems, vague uneasy sensations or pain pertaining to their abdomen, head, etc.), and even suicidal ruminations or urges.

When such adolescents report suicidal ruminations or urges, their reports have to be taken seriously, especially because these adolescents have a history of conduct problems and "manipulative behavior," and hence, many professionals would have a natural resistance to taking their complaints seriously and empathizing with them. At times–though infrequently-, one may observe a full-blown depressive episode, even with accompanying hallucinations and delusions. The hallucinations and delusions, when they occur, are usually congruent with their depressed mood, accompanied by urgings or beliefs that they have committed something sinful or bad and, deserve to die or that they are suffering from some terrible and incurable illness, etc.

Auditory Hallucinations

As mentioned in the section on pre-pubertal children also, contrary to popular belief that most adolescents who experience auditory hallucinations are suffering from schizophrenia, the fact is that most such adolescents, actually, may be suffering from bipolar disorder.[24] Auditory hallucinations can occur in several contexts in the adolescent who is experiencing bipolar disorder, especially with the atypical variety we have been discussing. Such youngsters who are intensely emotional because of the bipolar disorder, often report, that they experience their own "mind" or a "voice" in their "head" or "brain" "talking" to them or urging them to do one thing or another. They experience such hallucinatory type of phenomena, usually, when they are in an intense emotional state, such as being very angry with some one or when engaged in a physical altercation or fight. On such occasions, they may hear a voice urging them to fight, hurt the other person, etc. When depressed or intensely unhappy, they may hear a voice urging them to end their life. On the other hand, when they are in a state of excitation with manic or hypomanic features they may hear their "mind" or a "voice" in their head say, that they should go ahead and "have fun," "don't listen" to the teacher, etc. They tend to behave in an unruly and disruptive manner when experiencing such phenomena. Such youngsters often report that they have difficulty resisting these voices or urgings. Adolescents who are experiencing such hallucinatory phenomena are often experiencing a worsening of their illness. During such periods, their behavior and functioning deteriorate, and they behave in an overactive, impulsive, aggressive, and generally unruly manner. At times they mention a struggle between good and bad in their head or "brain." They experience voices or commands representing evil ("the devil") arguing or tussling with those representing goodness ("God" or "angel")—one urging them to be "bad" and the other prompting them to be "good." When they are predominantly in a depressive phase, the voices or urgings have a negative or depressive connotation. Usually the voices make negative remarks about them, such as "You are stupid," "You are ugly," etc., or urge them to end their lives. Many youngsters say or divulge very little, spontaneously, when interviewed during such states. However, on probing gently, they often reveal such experiences, or acknowledge the voices urging them not to talk or divulge information to others–a reason why such youngsters are often difficult to interview and understand.

Though, understandably, most adolescents are uneasy or guarded when acknowledging or divulging information about such hallucinatory experiences, many state somewhat casually that they have heard voices for many years, starting from their childhoods. When the voices are not very intense or distressing and have been an ongoing experience for quite sometime, the youngsters appear to take a matter of fact approach to them. Often, the thoughts or conflicts that underlie such voices are fairly evident. As in adults, the auditory hallucinations and related phenomena have a graded quality to them in adolescents (and children) also.

The most benign of such experiences manifest, as the youngsters' own intense thought processes, perceived as coming from their own mind or brain. Hearing voices, about which they are not sure as to whether they are their own thinking or someone else's voice, seems to represent an intermediate sate of severity or pathology. **Voices that they experience as definitely coming from another person and, that make them behave in an** abnormal manner, represent the most severe form of such phenomena. Youngsters who experience such severe forms of auditory hallucinations are in an intense state of the illness and usually will require hospitalization, to prevent unfortunate happenings and to bring the abnormal phenomena in control, quickly.

Unlike the usual conviction of a schizophrenic person who may experience the voices as spoken by people real or imagined and about which they often lack insight, to a dangerous degree, the voices experienced by bipolar youngsters are often interpreted by them as coming from their own mind, brain, or head. When they are asked to point to, where they hear the voices or perceive them to be coming from, they, more often, point to their own head, as opposed to their ears or an outside source. They often state, "I know it is my own thinking," or "I know it is my own brain." A definite exception to this, are the youngsters who are in severe states of depression (depressive phase of bipolar illness) and who experience voices that appear so "real," accusing them of horrible deeds, or urging them to commit suicide–the urgings, at times being so powerful that they may try to end their lives, even through violent means. Such command hallucinations could completely obliterate any capacity for the youngsters to think objectively.

Visual Hallucinations

Visual hallucinations are much less frequent than auditory hallucinations in the atypical bipolar adolescents, but they do occur at times. They seem to experience visual hallucinations, or related abnormal visual phenomena in two separate contexts and intensities. The first one is, as part of an acute psychotic process occurring in the context of an intense, agitated depression, in which, they see frightening scenes, such as their house being on fire–experiences which send them into states of intense terror. In my experience, such frightening abnormal visual phenomena occur among bipolar adolescents when they are in a state of acute psychotic depression. *A sixteen year old girl who experienced such a frightening phenomena prior to her hospitalization, remarked months later when she was in a state of remission, "It was real, I really saw it," indicating how vivid the imagery was when it occurred.*

The second context, in which visual hallucinations or abnormal visual phenomena usually occur in bipolar youngsters, is of a more benign nature. Most common of these are the youngsters' reporting that they often see a relative who died—usually a grand parent who died and to whom they had an emotional bond. They state this in a matter-of-fact-manner. Asked how clearly they see the person, these youngsters often reply, "Just like you are sitting there." Some clinicians may describe such phenomena as "hysteric" in nature, but with our present lack of understanding of neurophysiological aspects of such phenomena, we cannot state definitely, what is a hysteric phenomenon and how it differs from a hallucinations.

Since bipolar disorder is an illness that confers high intensity to the emotionality and related perceptual experiences of the person affected by it, it is not surprising that those afflicted by it experience hallucinatory phenomena that depict their fears, concerns, conflicts, and longings.

Delusions

Delusions, which are essentially false and entrenched beliefs with little or no basis for them in reality, are not very common in the atypical form of bipolar disorder. In most circumstances, adolescents who profess delusional beliefs would be considered deranged, by their peers because their beliefs are so implausible to be true and are not part of the shared belief system of their community. In some cases the delusions would be outright bizarre. From this point of view, the atypical bipolar youngsters, generally, will not appear to be mentally ill–at least most of the time—to the average layperson. They do not usually express delusional beliefs. Most people consider them to be youngsters who have a very bad temper and "attitude," given to unruly behavior, and difficult, if not impossible to deal with. Though not delusional they can be very illogical in their arguments and demands, however.

Delusions, however, can occur for brief periods in these youngsters at times—usually during the worsening of their illness. Typically, when they are experiencing or exhibiting a period of increased excitability, elation, anger, irrationality, and related phenomena they may express thoughts or beliefs that are grandiose in nature. In this sense their symptomatology during those periods exhibit some features of classical mania or hypomania–an example of why the atypical bipolar disorder is very likely related to, or is a variant of classical bipolar disorder. Such grandiose beliefs usually involve ideas that they are very rich or famous or have super human capacities, etc.

A fourteen-year-old male, living with his single parent mother and several siblings and whose family was barely managing on social assistance, had been exhibiting severe problem behavior since early childhood. He had received diagnosis of ADHD from a very early age and had received, years of psychotherapy and treatment with stimulants, but was functioning poorly, going from one crisis situation, school suspension, or transfer from school to another. Very often the police had to be called into his apartment because of his anger control and related problems. In spite of being very intelligent he could never function in a regular class setting. During a period of worsening of his symptoms and behavior he had become irrationally demanding, insisting that his mother buy him one expensive object after another, in rapid succession. He was getting suspended from school, time and again, during this period. He was irrationally demanding and argumentative. When, this period of acute worsening subsided with treatment aimed at bipolar disorder, he stated: "I thought I was very rich…I thought mom should get me anything I asked for…I thought I could do anything I imagined…I thought I was superman…I had so much energy." He had a strong family history of bipolar disorder–including his own mother having the illness.

Classical forms of grandiose delusions, though uncommon in adolescents suffering from atypical bipolar disorder, can occasionally occur in the high energy, excited states in these children, but are much less common than in the manic states of classical bipolar disorder.

In the atypical bipolar disorder, delusions are, perhaps more likely to occur when the youngsters are in the depressive phase or are experiencing symptomatology of depression, which at times occur, in brief, more or less discrete episodes. Usually these delusions take the form of beliefs that they have committed sins for which they will be punished by God, that the police or peers are looking for them to harm them (there may be some basis in reality for these beliefs at times), that they are suffering from some serious illness (which at times is based on some minor physical problem or other), that they look "ugly," and others are laughing at them because of it (some youngsters stay homebound avoiding the outside world and school because of such beliefs), etc.

Obsessions and Compulsions

Obsessive-compulsive phenomena occur commonly in adolescents suffering from bipolar disorder. Though, perhaps it is more frequently observed to co-occur in those who suffer from more classical forms of bipolar disorder, it is not too uncommon in those suffering from the atypical type also. Whether the obsessive-compulsive symptoms are part and parcel of the bipolar problem itself or are a manifestation of a separate, but co-morbid condition, cannot be settled presently. My own biased opinion is that, it is a part of the bipolar problem itself. Not only is it common in bipolar illness, many youngsters who present with obsessive compulsive disorder, on closer examination, have underlying features of bipolar disorder and, often, a strong family history of bipolar disorder also. **It is understandable, as bipolar disorder is an illness of emotional intensity, and subsequently, those who suffer from it are more vulnerable to doubts they cannot ignore and, repetitively engage in attempts to ward off the anxiety and discomfort these doubts cause, by engaging in compulsive behaviors.** Because of the emotional over-sensitivity and intensity of feelings bipolar disorder causes in the sufferer, any doubt that comes to their mind tends to get "stuck", as they cannot shake off these doubts, like most others who are not so oversensitive and intense can. **These obsessive-compulsive phenomena tend to be more problematic when their mood is predominantly depressed, but can also occur as a persistent waxing and waning problem, even when depression is not a prominent feature.**

As mentioned at the beginning, it is not any one of the above-mentioned symptoms or phenomenon that, by it-self indicates the presence of atypical bipolar disorder. **Rather, it is the clustering of many of the above mentioned features in a waxing and waning manner that indicate, that this illness may be the cause for the turmoil in a particular adolescent's life.** An astute clinician, who detects the clustering of these phenomena and the undulating course of the problems, will be prompted to make further inquiries and ongoing observations, to confirm the presence bipolar disorder, when it is likely to be the root-cause of the adolescent's problems.

Even though, recent writings on childhood and adolescent bipolar disorder mention mixed and rapid cycling forms of the illness, as perhaps, the most common presentation of bipolar disorder in children and adolescents, in my experience, the most common presentation is the one that we just discussed—the atypical bipolar disorder. **Intense temperament, aggression, anger control problems, excitability, hyperactivity, impulsivity, over-emotionality, over-reactivity, explosiveness, irritability, dysphoria, depression, obsessive compulsive problems, eating disorders, sleep problems, and others mentioned above intertwine to a problematic degree in this form of bipolar disorder. Occasionally, clearly identifiable episodes of depression and, at times, elation to a hypomanic level, during which behavioral problems predominate also occur.** Such adolescents, rarely if ever, attain a lasting, stable state or period of full remission of their symptomatology.

With the atypical bipolar disorder, the easily identifiable bipolar features, if they occur, are masked by the adolescent's turmoil prone and uneven existence, making it difficult for those who are not well aware of the nature and significance of those manifestations, to identify the illness.

The true nature of these adolescents' problems: the atypical bipolar dis-order—can only be confirmed by a painstaking, comprehensive evalua-tion and observations on an ongoing basis. In many youngsters, it may take several months—even a year or more, of knowing the youngster and his problems well, to confirm the diagnosis. However, clinicians who are well aware of this disorder and its complex manifestations will almost always encounter enough information during the initial evaluation itself, to strongly suspect that the youngster's problems may be due to atypical bipolar disorder.

CHAPTER V

ETIOLOGY OF BIPOLAR DISORDER: A BRIEF INTRODUCTION

Though the main purpose in writing this book is to bring about greater awareness of the widespread, yet unrecognized occurrence of bipolar disorder in children, a brief and introductory discussion on the etiology of this illness may be relevant. This chapter is intended, only for those who have very little or no knowledge of what is known about the etiology of this illness presently.

Almost all clinicians and researchers, who have good knowledge of bipolar disorder, are convinced that bipolar disorder is essentially a genetic illness. In almost all instances of this illness occurring in children, careful history taking and observations will reveal that, at least one parent, and some blood relatives going back generations have been affected by the illness, in one form or another. In the case of some young children, their parents—especially if they themselves are very young—may not have gone through the age period when the illness is most likely to manifest, and hence, may appear not to be affected by it. Often, only subtle manifestations of the illness may be evident in the parent. Only careful history taking and knowing the parent or parents well, over a period of time, in the clinical context will it become evident if there are significant features of bipolar disorder evident. At times, neither parent may be exhibiting significant features of this illness, but history and, or, observations of the grand parents will reveal either a clear picture, or subtle, but convincing evidence of this illness affecting previous generations. Keep in mind, always, however, that just because a parent or close blood relatives are affected by this illness, it does not automatically make the child's problems also a manifestation of bipolar disorder.

In this connection, **it is wise to remember also that, bipolar disorder is not an all-or-none phenomenon. People are affected by various gradations of intensity of this illness.** Some people may experience and exhibit a severe temperament and occasional spells of mild depression only and, may get by in life, usually, as difficult people to deal with. Only those who know such people really well may know how troubled, difficult, or dysfunctional they may or may not be. Many lead successful lives. Many can be productive, for periods of time–even extremely productive. Often, they are endowed with superior intelligence, which can compensate for some of their glaring temperamental and emotional problems—at least in the work setting. Many, if not most, never seek or receive psychiatric treatment. This does not mean they are not ill. Many parents, of bipolar children who come into treatment, belong to this category–affected by bipolar disorder and significantly dysfunctional because of it, but seldom identified as such or admitting to having psychiatric problems. Many parents, even seriously affected by the illness, refuse psychiatric treatment.

In this sense, bipolar disorder may be similar to illnesses such as rheumatoid arthritis, in the variable intensity with which it manifests in people. Some people are only mildly affected by an illness such as rheumatoid arthritis and can get by with an occasional analgesic or anti-inflammatory medicine, but some are crippled by it even from a young age, failing to respond sufficiently to all treatment available.

Given the fact, that this illness often occurs in a subtle manner in the children and their close blood relatives, obtaining family history that indicates the manifestations and presence of this disorder is extremely important in the identification of it. Because this illness often appears in parents and other close family members with only subtle manifestations, clinicians face a difficult task in trying to elicit family history indicative of bipolar disorder. Hence, the task requires special skills and awareness.

Taking a family history or conducting observations to identify this disorder in parents and close blood relatives is a difficult and sensitive issue. Parents understandably are frightened at the prospect that their children–and even they—are, or may be, affected by this disorder. Their fear and anger at such a prospect, often, make them deny, withhold, or distort crucial information that points to the presence of this illness in them, their children, or other family members. Moreover, their anger and anxiety related to these issues, often, are projected on to the clinician, who may be suspecting that the child and even other family members may be suffering from a serious psychiatric illness such as this. Parents, often, would rather believe that the children's or their own problems are justified reactions to environmental problems—often their response to the unjust or troublesome behavior of others. Though, at times, there may be some truth to such environmental problems playing a precipitating or perpetuating role, the fact, that the reactions or problems manifest in the form of this illness, rather than anything else, points to their underlying biological vulnerability to this illness. Since, such insights are frightening and extremely guilt producing for the parents—though it is clearly not due to any fault of theirs–, often, they will not be very cooperative in identifying this illness in their children. They also resist pharmacological treatment for the children to address this illness, the treatment, even though not curative, may at least be helpful to a degree.

These problems are compounded by the fact that many professionals involved in the care of such children, lack the capacity to detect and deal with this illness, or are prejudiced against such a diagnosis due to professional or personal reasons. Parents use such resistance or lack of awareness in the professionals and the subsequent misinformation they give the parents about the child's problems, to fortify their own resistance to such a diagnosis. Added to these difficulties is the fact that treatment of bipolar disorder is still very unsatisfactory, even in adults—and more unsatisfactory in children. The inadequacy of treatment available presently, is especially glaring in our inability to bring about full and lasting remission of the illness and in preventing relapses.

Though, it is quite evident that bipolar disorder is biological in origin, and genetic in most cases (except perhaps in cases where there have been reports of bipolar type of symptomatology manifesting in adults due to brain injury or infections), the exact genetic and biochemical causes of this disorder are still quite unclear. Genetic studies have shown linkage to several chromosomes, including chromosomes 4, 6, 11, 18, 21, and X.[4,13,16,20,25,30,34,38] Recent studies have pointed to possible association between bipolar disorder and serotonin (5HT) activity regulating genes.[18,38] Recently, serotonin receptor gene polymorphism in mitochondrial D.N.A., as a possible cause of bipolar disorder, via alteration of brain energy metabolism, was implicated as a possible cause of this disorder.[25] However, these studies have not been conclusively replicated, and the gene or genes that are responsible for bipolar disorders are yet to be identified in a fully convincing manner. The fact that several chromosomes and regions have been implicated does not mean that these studies are flawed. Most clinicians and researchers, at present, are of the opinion that bipolar disorders are a group of disorders with many manifestations that are common for the group and other manifestations that are unique to one sub-group compared to others. Such a concept will account for the genetic heterogeneity, at least to a degree. In this connection, it is helpful to note, that the most commonly used official diagnostic manual,[2] uses the term Bipolar Disorders (not bipolar disorder), acknowledging that, there are various forms of this disorder or illness. The subcategory Bipolar Disorder NOS[20] listed under the heading Bipolar Disorders, and the diagnostic category Mood disorder NOS, are acknowledgements, that there are forms of bipolar and related mood disorders that cannot be clearly categorized presently using the methods available. When I come across the multitude of children affected by atypical forms of bipolar disorder in my day-to-day work, I am forced to rely on the categories Bipolar Disorder NOS and Mood Disorder NOS, often, as official diagnostic categories, fully cognizant of the fact that these terms and what they vaguely represent are inadequate, to effectively convey the type of problems these children suffer from. I hope, the day will soon come, when a more definitive method to diagnose and categorize bipolar disorders will occur, as a result of research efforts using modern biotechnology.

Clinicians and researchers have been identifying various subgroups and categories of bipolar disorders, in addition to those that are presently acknowledged in the official diagnostic manuals. The term Bipolar Spectrum Disorders now commonly used by experts in the field of bipolar disorders in adults, points to the clinical and genetic heterogeneity of this disorder,[1,6] significantly beyond what has been acknowledged in the diagnostic manuals. Though the various subgroups of the disorder–the ones officially acknowledged, the ones newly identified, the atypical bipolar disorder in children and adolescents we have discussed in previous chapters, etc., may have genetic and biochemical similarities, obviously there are differences also to account for the varied clinical manifestations. The variable response to treatment measures also point to an underlying biochemical heterogeneity. **The fact that these disorders most often present as episodic or waxing and waning, points to biochemical factors that periodically go out of control in one form or another, rather than permanent structural abnormalities of the brain, causing these disorders.** Until the abnormal genetic and biochemical mechanisms, which cause the illness and control its course are well understood, fully effective treatment measures are almost impossible to develop. Until the biochemical abnormalities concerned can be detected through laboratory measures in a valid and reliable manner, the diagnosis of this illness will have to solely depend on clinical observations and history gathering, as at present.

Though there are reasons to believe that several neurotransmitter aberrations may be involved in producing the manifestations of this illness, none has been conclusively proven to be causative. The fact that the diagnosis of bipolar illness is, still, entirely based on clinical observations and history, attest to that fact. For quite some time there have been reports from brain imaging research studies conducted, of various abnormalities in brain structure or function of people (research subjects) suffering from bipolar disorder. Again, such findings have not been conclusively replicated in a reliable or practical manner and do not have much application in the diagnosis and treatment of this illness at present. Such investigations and measures remain at research level only and are not yet useful in identifying, or ruling out this illness in a particular individual, for clinical purposes. However, it is only through such research efforts using modern biological tools and technology that better identification and treatment of the illness will come about, and hence, a brief discussion of some of the present research efforts to understand the underlying mechanisms of the illness, is appropriate.

Since the 1960s dysregulation of monoamine neurotransmitters–norepinehrine, dopamine, and serotonin-, have been considered to play a crucial role in producing the manifestations of bipolar disorder. Though a great deal of research has been done to clarify the roles and mechanisms of monoamine actions in bipolar disorder, the exact mechanisms and roles they play continue to be unclear. At present, most researchers consider these neurotransmitters, either alone, or combined, or in concert with other neurotransmitters or biochemical factors to play a crucial role in the manifestations of bipolar disorder.

Abnormalities in cyclic-adenosine-monophosphate (cAMP) mechanisms are considered to play a role in the manifestations of this illness and have been an avenue of recent research explorations.[12, 31] Regulation abnormalities of G proteins, as a possible causative factor, have been another area of recent research.[3, 28] Monoamine signaling variations and its effect on hypothalamic-adrenal-axis functioning in producing the symptomatology of bipolar disorder has been an area of interest for quite some time. The new technologies in molecular biology and brain imaging are expected to make such studies much more effective.[27]

The use of brain imaging, as a tool in diagnosing and conducting research to clarify the etiology and improve the treatment of bipolar disorder is bound to increase with the advancing technology in brain imaging. The new techniques in brain imaging which do not require exposure to radiation may become an effective tool in the study of bipolar disorder.[37] Structural brain imaging has demonstrated white matter hyper-intensities [37] in people suffering from bipolar disorder. Spectroscopic studies have given evidence of possible abnormalities in the metabolism of choline containing compounds in symptomatically ill bipolar patients.[37] Decreased activity of the prefrontal cortex in bipolar patients during the depressive phase has been demonstrated by blood flow and metabolic studies.[37] Anterior cingulate and amygdala have also been implicated in the pathophysiology of bipolar disorder.[27] The significance of the reported findings from brain imaging studies is not well understood however.[37] Researchers using brain imaging, as a tool to investigate the etiology and treatment of bipolar disorder, feel very optimistic that the field has a very promising future.[37]

Goals for research in bipolar disorder, recently articulated from the National Institute of Mental Health,[20] offer hope that the importance of research in elucidating the etiology and improving treatment of this disorder (at least in adults), is perhaps beginning to get some of the much needed attention. However, it also makes clear, how little we know and how much more has to be done before the devastation caused by this illness and the hopelessness it creates come to an end.

Without knowing the genetic and biochemical mechanisms that cause this illness, fully effective remedies are difficult, if not impossible, to develop. Unless the community-at-large become aware, how common this illness is among all age groups, especially children, and how devastating its effects are to the individual, family, and society and, of the urgent manner in which financial and other resources have to be dedicated to combat this genetic disease, the devastation caused by this illness will only worsen for generations to come.

Chapter VI

Treatment of Bipolar Disorder in Children: Some general guidelines

At the outset, I would like to make it clear that this chapter or book is not intended as a guide to treatment of bipolar disorder in children. I have mentioned, time and again, my opinion, that the treatment available for this disorder presently, especially for children, is extremely inadequate. One of the purposes of writing this book, is to stimulate more awareness that research to develop better remedies for this disorder is urgently needed, by pointing out how prevalent yet unrecognized this illness is and how inadequate the remedies available today are.

This chapter is only a general, introductory discussion and critique of treatment of bipolar disorder in children. People familiar with the treatment available for this disorder today, such as psychiatrists and related professionals, may not find much that is new in this chapter and hence, may skip reading this chapter, if they so prefer.

Once bipolar disorder is strongly suspected or confirmed in a child, as best as one can, the question arises as to what could be done for the child concerned. Given the limitations of treatments available today and the imperfect results they produce—even in adults, for whom these treatments were first developed-, and given the fact that they are, perhaps, even less useful for children, the issue of treatment for this disorder in children remains a great concern.

Before discussing the issue of treatment further, one point needs emphasis. **Bipolar disorder in children–especially the atypical forms–occur in all** gradations of severity, as is the case for this illness in adults also. An experienced psychiatrist can detect this illness in many children, but the degree to which the illness affects the children vary considerably. Some children may exhibit problem behavior or experience troublesome symptomatology only to a mild degree or only occasionally. In contrast, some children may remain severely troubled by the illness most of their life. The intensity and persistence with which the illness affects their lives have to be given important consideration in making the decision, as to whether, and when, treatment is needed, what type of treatment, the duration of it, etc. The children who are only mildly affected may require only minimal interventions, and that too, often, for short durations only, compared to those more severely affected. Remember, one is not treating an illness, but rather the occurrence of the illness, in varying severity, in a particular child. Many adults with bipolar disorder, who are only mildly affected by this illness, are able to live very productive lives with minimal treatment or supportive measures. This is true of children also.

Always keep in mind that a vast number of children may be affected by this illness, but some, luckily, may be affected only to a mild degree. My experience suggests that, it is probably the group of children who are affected by less severe forms of the illness, who may appear to benefit from treatment with stimulants, when they are given such treatment because of the belief that they are suffering from ADHD. Some, or many such children only mildly affected by the illness, may be able to get by with other, supportive, or intermittent interventions also.

However, the very fact that bipolar disorder starts manifesting in some children at a very young age, suggests, that the tendency for this disorder—most likely the genetic vulnerability to it—is unusually strong in these children. Another possibility is that the genetic vulnerability is acted upon adversely by the environmental problems impacting on these children's lives, making the illness surface at a young age. A word of caution is in order here, however. The chaotic circumstances of many of these children's lives, on closer scrutiny, are often due to the effects of bipolar disorder in a parent or parents. For example, parents who suffer from this disorder are prone to a life of chaos because of the very nature of this illness. Their chaotic existence affects others around them also, especially their children. Parents suffering from this illness are more prone to divorce, being single parents, unemployment, financial ruin, drug and alcohol abuse, violence, or to just leading a highly disorganized and seemingly irresponsible life style that affects their family members, especially children, in a seriously adverse manner. In this sense, the children who are genetically vulnerable to bipolar disorder, face a double jeopardy: the adverse effects of their genetic liability and the adverse effects caused by the parents who suffer from the illness. These complex sets of circumstances, in turn, adversely interfere with the treatment of these children also. For example, often, parents suffering from the illness are temperamentally unstable, prone to irrational thinking and becoming agitated, explosive, and over-anxious. In spite of the psychiatrist's best efforts, they refuse to cooperate with their children's treatment in any reasonable manner and will not allow the child to receive appropriate treatment. Such parents, often, are unable to accept that their children are affected by a serious mental illness. This is a problem that most parents of bipolar children exhibit to some degree, but in the parents suffering from the illness, become such a complex and intense issue-, which, interacting with their (parents') biological vulnerabilities and psychological concerns assume a formidable, if not impossible impediment to the treatment of children.

Most parents—even those with adequate or superior coping skills—will require the utmost of care, support, and understanding to come to terms with the diagnosis of bipolar disorder in their children, and the clinicians have to have special understanding and capacity to help the parent through the extremely trying circumstances. **The devastation that a diagnosis of bipolar disorder in their child can produce in parents should never be minimized.**

Parents, often express anger at the clinician for seriously entertaining the possibility of such an illness in their children. They may break off treatment, go through various phases of denial, attribute the manifestations of the illness as justified reactions to environmental stresses only, or to teen-age problems. Parents who are divorced, separated, or in serious conflict with each other, often perceive their children's problems, only as reactions to the behavior and problems of the other parent.

The diagnosis of bipolar disorder in a child, often subjects the diagnosing clinician to a spate of adverse reactions and challenges from the parents. These are trying circumstances for the clinician and would require his or her utmost patience, objectivity, and equanimity to maintain or salvage a reasonably positive treatment relationship with the parents. Such trying circumstances and negative emotional reactions to which they become the target of, often dissuade clinicians from diagnosing bipolar disorder in children—especially in out patient settings. Because of these reasons and the reasons mentioned earlier, clinicians often fail to venture beyond diagnoses of ADHD, other disruptive disorders,[2] or depression when dealing with seriously, behaviorally and emotionally disturbed children.

Diagnosing and treating bipolar disorder in children, especially in the out patient settings, is an extremely demanding, time consuming, and emotionally draining venture that requires strong commitment by the treating psychiatrist. The financial remuneration, especially in today's managed care environment, is often severely inadequate to compensate for the time and effort needed and the stress involved. This means, that motivations other than monetary remuneration are needed to treat such youngsters effectively, on an ongoing basis. The very nature of the illness makes many, if not most youngsters, hostile and less than cooperative. Many psychiatrists and clinicians simply lack the motivation and stamina to effectively deal with these youngsters or their parents. Because of the multiple problems involved and the crisis proneness of these youngsters, a highly committed clinic setting, attached or affiliated to a hospital that has psychiatric emergency room and in patient admission facilities for children of all ages, is the best venue for treating the bipolar youngsters on an ongoing basis. Many of these youngsters would require periodic short-term hospitalizations, and some may need long-term residential placement.

Since the treatment available today is less than satisfactory for many, if not the majority of people–adults and children—who suffer from bipolar disorder, in spite of best treatment efforts, a significant proportion, if not the majority of people, who suffer from the more severe forms of this disorder continue to suffer immensely and lead very troubled lives. Only very limited progress, if any, has occurred in the treatment of this disorder during the past quarter of a century. Any new medicines that have been approved for the treatment of this disorder have not substantially altered the treatment outcome compared to that of twenty-five years back. However, the sensational news reports—especially on television, which occur periodically-, and the claims of drug companies, may make one believe that once a person starts taking the medicines touted, the bipolar problem would just go away or diminish to one of minor inconvenience only. Nothing could be farther from the truth. If such is the state of affairs with adults, the plight of children who suffer from this illness is even worse.

Overall, treatment for this disorder available today helps, significantly, less than half of the people treated. Even they are burdened by problematic side effects, and a good majority of them discontinue treatment because of side effects or concerns about them or because of their perception that the treatment is not sufficiently beneficial. At present, majority of the adults severely affected by bipolar disorder, are unable to live an independent life or work and earn a living, in spite of the best treatment efforts. Many children, who are in treatment with presently available medicines and other treatments, are still unable to function well in school or home. Side effects of medicines and incomplete symptom remission interfere with their academic functioning and progress. Many adults and children continue to be symptomatic and lead unsettled, troubled, troublesome, and crisis prone lives. A majority of adults and children seriously affected by this illness are unable to lead anything close to a normal life, in spite of the best treatment efforts.

Because of above-mentioned facts, **this illness should get the priority and attention it deserves as one of the most devastating challenges confronting humanity. In my opinion, it is second only to AIDS in the urgency and attention it deserves as a medical, public health, and social problem.**

Prior to the 1970s neuroleptics or anti-psychotics (a poor term of course), tricyclic antidepressants, and Electro Convulsive Therapy (ECT), were the main treatments available for bipolar disorder. In the early 1970s, lithium carbonate became available, mainly for the treatment of mania and as maintenance treatment to prevent recurrences of mania. About twenty-five years passed before another anti-manic (and possibly mood stabilizing) drug—valproic acid—was approved for the treatment of this condition. Whether valproic acid is significantly more effective than lithium, is still being debated. However, one thing is clear: most bipolar patients, who take these medicines, continue to be symptomatic or experience relapses. However, having several pharmacological options to treat the illness–inadequate as each one may be-, is indeed an improvement, as many people respond to one medicine better than the other, or may not tolerate one medicine for one reason or another. Moreover, bipolar disorders, being a group that contains several related disorders, most likely, are caused by related, but not exactly the same genetic and biochemical mechanisms. Because of the heterogeneity of the underlying mechanisms, in order to effectively control the manifestations of these illnesses, several medicines that act through different mechanisms may be needed to effectively deal with them.

Bipolar disorders pose several challenges in treatment. The fact that the illness has, in many cases, two distinct phases—mania and depression, and in other cases, varying manifestations such as mixed phases, unremitting symptomatology, predominance of anger and irritability (rather than elation and depression), co-occurrence of hallucinations, delusions, and other symptomatology such as manifestations of anxiety, obsessions, compulsions, etc., makes it very unlikely that the same pharmacological agents or combinations would succeed in varying groups and in varying phases. For example, neuroleptics may control mania, but they will not prevent and are not primary treatment agents for the depressive phase of the illness. In fact, some neuroleptics may even induce or worsen depression. This is understandable, if one considers mania and depression representing opposite poles of the bipolar illness, with increased energy being a characteristic of mania and anergy the hallmark of bipolar depression. It is logical to conclude that the biochemical mechanisms underlying mania has to be quite different from or the opposite of that causing depression. Similarly antidepressants are not effective in treating the manic phase of the illness and may even precipitate or worsen manic episodes.

Lithium and valproic acid are primarily anti-manic drugs, and they, to an extent, help prevent the recurrence of manic episodes. However, they have only limited beneficial effect, if any, in the depressive phase and in preventing recurrence of depression. In addition, antidepressants—including the selective serotonin reuptake inhibitors (SSRIs)—that are quite effective in unipolar depressions, are not as effective in the depressive phase of bipolar illness. Also, no antidepressant is free from the tendency to induce mania. All this points to the treatment of bipolar disorder being a complex and daunting endeavor, even in adults, and even more challenging in children.

The treatment of bipolar disorder in children requires great deal of experience in the assessment of symptomatology and in fine-tuning the complex medication regimens. The aim is to maintain optimal improvement, while keeping the side effects to a minimum. This includes, long-term adverse effects of the medicines on the growing child and enabling the child to function as effectively as possible at home and school.

There are several guidelines, which summarize the presently available pharmacological treatments for bipolar disorder. Most of these deal primarily with treatment of adults, with some references to children. Essentially, the same pharmacological agents used for adults are used for children also, but in smaller doses. Hence the guidelines for adults are helpful with children also, though, some of the experimental or "off label" use (use in conditions other than those they have been approved for) of medicines in adults, such as the newer anticonvulsants lamotrigine, topiramate, etc., are best avoided in children until more information becomes available about their effectiveness and safety in bipolar disorder. An excellent summary of medication treatment available today for bipolar disorder can be found in the publication "Medication treatment of Bipolar Disorder 2000." [36]

The fact that every new anticonvulsant, neuroleptic, or antidepressant which come into the market is given a try in the treatment of bipolar disorder, is proof of how psychiatrists feel that the presently available remedies are inadequate and how desperately they hope that something else could turn out to be more effective. It also reveals that the treatment of bipolar disorder is still at a very uncertain stage.

In general, it is better to be cautious and conservative in the use of medicines in treating bipolar disorder in children. Use medicines that have a long "track record" of being effective and having a very favorable side effect profile. Any off label use of medicines should be undertaken, only, when the more conventional and approved remedies have failed, taking appropriate precautions and informing the parents (and youngsters also, in an appropriate manner) why they are being recommended and what adverse effects everyone need to be aware of.

With the above cautionary statements as backdrop, the following discussion on treatment of bipolar disorder in children may be helpful for those whose experience in the matter is limited. The ideas expressed here are based primarily on my experience only and are not intended as a definitive guide to the treatment of bipolar disorder in children. Psychiatrists and others with good deal of experience in the treatment of bipolar disorder in children may not gain much by reading this chapter, as it is not intended for those with such experience and hence, may want to skip reading this chapter, if they so desire.

Treatment of bipolar disorder in children, in general, may pose more complex challenges than treatment of the illness in adults. To start with, the disorder, often, is more difficult to diagnose in children. In some cases, it will take many months or even a few years before the psychiatrist concerned could safely conclude that a child's problems are definitely due to bipolar disorder. Bipolar disorder, as mentioned before, more often than not, presents in a complex and atypical manner. One has to always take into consideration the opinions and fears of the youngsters and parents as to what the nature of the problem may be. Parents, for understandable reasons, are always reluctant to subject the children to anything other than the smallest dose possible of the least toxic of the medicines. Sometimes, even for years, they will refuse to give the child any medicine intended for the illness, because of fear and stigma. Children–especially, adolescents–are often reluctant or refuse to take medicines intended to improve their behavior. Even if they take the medicines when the problems are severe, they soon stop or oppose taking them, as they feel they are better and can do without them or because of side effects. Many children "hate" or are afraid of blood tests or totally refuse to submit to blood tests that are required for taking the medicines.

Most adults who suffer from severe forms of bipolar disorder are not able to work and usually receive disability or other benefits. In contrast, children who are severely affected by this illness are still expected to get up early (at times painfully too early) every morning and go to school regularly–some times for all twelve months of the year-, cope with school and homework, keep their behavior and emotions in control, pass the required examinations, etc.,–all difficult, if not impossible tasks for them. These problems are compounded by the fact that they have to take medicines that have side effects, which often make them drowsy and interfere with their capacities. Such challenges and special problems require special understanding and experience with the pharmacotherapy and overall treatment of bipolar disorders in children.

The ideas expressed below are based on my experience in dealing with the above mentioned and related issues, while trying to be of help to bipolar children and their caregivers during the past three decades.

The Treatment Setting

If a youngster is found to be suffering from bipolar disorder, the treatment will be influenced by the setting in which it occurs and other factors. These factors include the willingness or not of the child and parents to accept psychopharmacological treatment and specifically, the medicines recommended by the psychiatrist. Psychopharmacological treatment, also depends on how reliable the youngsters are in taking the medicines, how reliable the parents are in administering them regularly, the age of the youngster, how definite the diagnosis appears to be, whether classical or atypical features predominate, the phase of the illness, the need and willingness to adhere to any blood monitoring that may be needed with certain medicines, and related factors. The fact that youngsters suffering from even severe manifestations of the illness are expected to function in school and cope with the school demands, also would influence treatment efforts, the types of medicines used, dosages, time of administration, etc.

Let us first examine the common scenarios in initiating and maintaining out patient treatment with the bipolar youngsters. Most often when treatment aimed at bipolar disorder become necessary, the youngsters are between the ages 8-18. Usually they have a long history of highly problematic behavior that has not responded, well enough, and consistently, to psychotherapeutic measures and treatment with stimulant medicines (Ritalin, Dexedrine, etc.). Let us assume that, a very likely or definite diagnosis of bipolar disorder has been arrived upon by careful evaluation and observation over a period of time. Most of these youngsters may have had a past diagnosis of ADHD. Often, the younger children will be continuing to take stimulant medication at the time the diagnosis is made. If the youngsters are in an acute state of worsening of symptomatology or behavior, with severe behavioral dyscontrol or frank signs of mania, or is in a state of severe depression, a decision has to be made whether the child is best treated in an inpatient setting. Unless the child is exhibiting florid mania or psychosis, or features of severe depression with definite suicide risk are present, most parents are reluctant to consider in patient treatment, especially if the child has not had prior psychiatric inpatient admission(s). After explaining to the parents that the psychiatrist is strongly recommending in patient admission—if such a measure appears to be indicated-, often, because of the reluctance of the parents and child to accept in patient treatment and due to other impediments the psychiatrist may have little choice but to treat the child as an out patient. Other than refusal by the youngster and parents, the usual impediments for in patient treatment are the reluctance or refusal by insurance companies to authorize hospitalization, the refusal of many hospitals to admit youngsters exhibiting behavior problems and aggression or keep them there for sufficient time until they are well enough to be treated as out patients, etc. If the child is not posing an imminent danger to his own life in a manner that is evident to most everyone, very often, the psychiatrist may have little choice but to initiate or continue treatment in the out patient setting itself, unless a for-profit hospital is available that may admit the child using less stringent criteria. Of course there is the ever-present problem of many youngsters not having medical insurance for hospitalization, which frustrates many who work in low-income areas. In my experience, today, most bipolar youngsters end up being treated as outpatients, even during acute episodes, because of above mentioned impediments to in patient admission.

If a child is in manic, hypo-manic, or mixed state or is in a state with severe behavioral dyscontrol and aggression as predominant features–as it often happens with children suffering from atypical bipolar disorder—and the child is on stimulant medication, the first step to undertake is to discontinue it, because of the strong possibility that stimulant medicines induce or worsen such states. After making sure the physical health of the child and baseline laboratory measures do not contraindicate any particular medicine to be used, the child could be started on small doses of an atypical neuroleptic such as risperidone. The initial dose selected is in the range of 0.5 to 1 mg. once or twice a day, to be titrated upwards carefully every two to three days by increments of 0.5 to 1 mg a day (note that the use of risperidone in mania or hypomania without delusions or hallucinations is an off label use presently, but one which has clinically proven to be quite effective and well tolerated in general). Keep in mind that medicines such as risperidone may induce dystonic reactions even in small doses in some youngsters. If the child is sleeping poorly and is remaining excited and disruptive at night use of diphenhydramine (12.5 mg to 25mg) or hydroxyzine (10 to 25 mg) could be helpful until the acute excitement and high-energy state—which underlies the sleep problem-, abates. Benzodiazepines, especially lorazepam or clonazepam in 0.5–2mg. dose at bed time is also very useful to provide sleep and rest in acute excited states, but one has to keep in mind their habit forming potential, especially in many adolescents who may already have shown a tendency to abuse drugs. **Withholding such medicines from adolescents routinely or without sufficient reason–just because adolescents are considered a high-risk group for drug abuse-, is not at all correct or ethical, however.**

The youngster should be seen two or three times a week during this initial phase of treatment and the parents should have liberal access to the psychiatrist to consult on the phone regarding any concerns that may arise between visits. At each visit, assess progress, as per the reports of the child and parents and by mental status observations. Inquire and observe for any side effects of medicines. When the dose of risperidone reaches 2-3 mg. per day some children will be prone to neuromuscular side effects such as muscle rigidity, dystonia, and increased salivation. Inform the child and parents of such possibilities, so that they will not panic if any such phenomena emerge, but instead will report their concerns to the psychiatrist promptly. If such side effects emerge, they can be controlled by trihexphenidyl 1-4 mg. per day or benztropine 0.5—2 mg. per day. Efforts should be made to keep the dose of risperidone, below 3 mg per day in elementary school age children and below 6 mg per day in adolescents, as problematic side effects are more likely to occur above these doses. A small supply of one of the above-mentioned medicines to control side effects may be prescribed, to keep it handy, in case such side effects emerge. This will help allay the parents' and youngsters' fear of sudden emergence of side effects and being caught in a situation without having medicine at hand to control them.

Many children are reluctant to swallow pills and some adolescents may discard the medicines given them. In such situations liquid form of the medicine(s) may have to prescribed. One has to make sure the parents know how to measure out the correct dose of a medicine such as risperidone, which is marketed in 1mg. per mL dose. Often, a note to the pharmacist to demonstrate to the parent how exactly to measure out the correct dose, would be very helpful for the parent who feels uneasy and unsure of such measures, especially given the anxiety associated with starting a child on such medicines. Keeping in the office a sample bottle of the medicine(s) with the accompanying dropper, for demonstration purposes, is very helpful to demonstrate to the parents how to measure out the exact amount of the medicine, when prescribing such medicines for the first time.

Once measures such as above are instituted, the desirability of adding a mood regulator, such as divalproex or lithium carbonate also to the medication regimen has to be considered. (Some psychiatrists may prefer to start the child on a mood regulator as the first medicine to be started, but in my experience, it is more practical, especially in the out patient setting, to follow the sequence mentioned above.) Medicines, depicted as mood regulators have proven to be moderately helpful in the treatment of mania and in the prevention of relapses of it when used as a maintenance medicine (mainly for classical bipolar disorder). If the child's problems attain good control with the use of a neuroleptic such as risperidone, parents are often reluctant to give the child such mood regulators for prolonged periods, with their potential for toxicity, need for blood tests, etc. They usually agree for such measures, only if the simpler regimens fail to achieve remission or if relapses occur to a problematic degree.

The neuroleptic medicines that have been used commonly in youngsters, before the so-called atypical neuroleptics such as risperidone became available during the last several years were haloperidol and thioridazine. Recently, olanzapine, another atypical narcoleptic has also been coming into use, especially after it got approval from the Food and Drug Administration (FDA) for treatment of mania in adults.

Haloperidol, and thioridazine–to a lesser degree—have been used successfully in controlling mania, hypomania, and related behavioral and emotional dyscontrol problems in children, during the past three decades. Haloperidol, is equally, or more effective than risperidone in controlling the manic phase and related behavioral problems in children. Its main draw back is that it produces neuromuscular side effects such as tremor, rigidity, and dystonia even in small doses, in children and adolescents and is perhaps more prone to producing tardive dyskinesia on prolonged use. It may also induce the appearance of depressive phenomena in some children, if they are maintained on it much beyond the manic phase. However, if used carefully it can be very effective in bringing about resolution of acute manic symptoms or related severe behavioral dyscontrol, especially when other medicines prove ineffective or if the child's problems are so intense that an improvement has to be brought about quickly. The dose of haloperidol should be kept at the minimum possible, to minimize adverse effects. An appropriate starting dose for haloperidol in children and adolescents is 0.25 to 2 mg. per day, depending on the age and size of the youngster. Increase the dose carefully every two to three days. It is best to limit the daily dose to a maximum of 2 to 5mg. in elementary school age children, and below 10 mg per day with the adolescent age group. At doses above 1—2 mg. per day of haloperidol, it is wise to add trihexphenidyl 2-4 mg. per day or benztropine 0.5—2 mg. per day to prevent troublesome neuromuscular side effects, especially dystonia, which could be alarming for the child and parents if it occurs, and often makes them unwilling to continue the medicine. Keep in mind that dystonic side effects of neuroleptics occur more frequently in children and adolescents compared to adults.

Both risperidone and haloperidol (and most other neuroleptics) have a tendency to produce lactation in female adolescents because of such medicines' tendency to increase prolactin secretion. Some times simple reassurance would suffice in dealing with this problem, which is generally considered a benign side effect of neuroleptics, but if this fails to diminish the anxiety and objections of the adolescent or parents, a reduction in dosage or trial on another neuroleptic that is less likely to increase prolactin level, have to be undertaken. Generally, the tendency of a neuroleptic to block the effects of Dopamine 2 (D2) in the brain is positively correlated with its tendency to increase prolactin secretion and induce lactation. Even though atypical neuroleptics are considered weak D2 blockers, in practice, many of them also exhibit this adverse effect when administered to adolescents, for significant periods of time. At times, addition of small doses of bromocriptine, which reduces prolactin level and suppresses lactation, may be beneficial in ameliorating this problem.

Another useful neuroleptic, as mentioned above, to control manic excitement and related behavioral dyscontrol in children, especially if they are prone to neuromuscular side effects of neuroleptics, has been thioridazine, which rarely produces such problematic side effects in small doses. Because of its tendency to produce cardiac conduction problems, which have come into focus more and more recently, and the warning about this problem issued by Food and Drug Administration (FDA) recently, it is infrequently used in children at present. It can be quite effective in improving the aggressive, explosive behavior of atypical bipolar youngsters, if used judiciously and in small doses. Because of its tendency to cause cardiac conduction disorders, baseline and follow up electrocardiogram (EKG) monitoring is needed if this drug is to be prescribed. At present, thioridazine is to be prescribed, only if the more modern, atypical neuroleptics are not effective or are not tolerated for one reason or another. As per the guidelines presently recommended, if the QTc interval is above 500 milliseconds, thioridazine should not be given. Because of the above-mentioned problems, thioridazine may only be used very infrequently, if at all, in children from now on.

FDA has recently approved Olanzapine for the treatment of mania in adults. The effectiveness and feasibility of olanzapine–especially in long-term use–as an anti-manic drug, mood regulator, or in the control of bipolar disorder related behavior problems in children, is yet to be convincingly proven. Preliminary clinical experience suggests that as an anti-manic drug it may not be more effective than risperidone but may be, in general, as effective as many, if not most neuroleptics. Its tendency to produce significant weight gain (all neuroleptics in use in children, including risperidone, have this tendency, but medicines such as olanzapine may have a greater tendency to produce this side effect) may limit its usefulness for long-term use in youngsters. Adolescents especially, balk at taking it, once they know of, or notice the undesirable weight gain. It may have a role, however, in mania and related behavioral problems, especially when a youngster may not be able to tolerate other neuroleptics because of neuro-muscular side effects, as olanzapine rarely produces such side effects in small doses. When using this medicine in children (off label use), it is wise to start with 2.5 mg. per day and limit the dose to 5mg. per day in elementary-school-age children, and 10 mg. per day in the adolescent age group. Since there is only limited experience in the use of this medicine in very young children, it is wise to avoid its use in such age groups, at present. The reported side effects of this drug to increase blood sugar levels or precipitate diabetes should also be kept in mind. Olanzapine also produces prolactin increase and lactation in some female adolescents, though its reported mode of action suggests that it may be less likely to do so than haloperidol, risperidone, and many other neuroleptics that are more potent D2 blockers.

There is not enough experience with the use of quetiapine and ziprasidone (both atypical neuroleptics) in the treatment of bipolar disorder in children (or adults). Quetiapine's tendency to produce only minimal neuromuscular side effects and ziprasidone's reported benefit of not inducing weight gain, calls for careful studies in their use in bipolar disorder, starting with adults. If they prove to be beneficial in bipolar disorder in adults, use in children will inevitably follow. Ziprasidone's tendency to produce cardiac conduction problems and the need for EKG monitoring at baseline and periodically, has to be kept in mind when it is used.

Mood regulators such as valproic acid and lithium carbonate are introduced in the acute phase of mania or as maintenance treatment to prevent relapses, if the parents and youngsters are amenable to the use of such medicines and are willing to adhere to the need for blood tests required, prior to starting treatment and while being maintained on them. The psychiatrist has a better chance of convincing the parents to give their child a trial on such medicines, if signs of classical mania occur, are severe, and the parents are convinced that the child suffers from a serious mental illness. When features of mania deviate from the classical form or when behavioral and anger problems predominate (as in atypical bipolar disorder), parents and others often continue to interpret the child's problems as bad behavior rather than as a manifestation of a serious illness. In such situations, only after several months or years of troubled and troublesome behavior, relapses, or treatment failures will many parents become convinced that a trial on such medicines is worth the risk. Many parents and youngsters agree for treatment with mood regulators, but discontinue it when the acute problems subside. Added to these problems is the fact that effectiveness of these medicines, especially in atypical bipolar disorder, and to an extend in the classical variety also, is less than what is required and hoped for, and many parents and youngsters may want much more than what these medicines can provide for them.

Divalproex, which is a derivative of valproic acid and produces less gastrointestinal adverse effects than the parent compound, is often the first mood regulator tried today, though, lithium carbonate may be equally or more effective in many children. Except in very young children—who are more vulnerable to the hepatic toxicity of divalproex-, it is somewhat easier to maintain children on this medicine, compared to lithium, because of its wider margin of safety. A reasonable starting dose for divalproex is 125 mg. twice a day in younger children and 250 mg. twice a day in the adolescent age group. The dose can be adjusted upwards every few days, depending on the blood level and how well the child is tolerating the medicine. The serum level is maintained between 50 to 125 Mcg./mL, which is considered the therapeutic level. Serum level of the drug and liver function are monitored closely, by blood tests, (about once in 1-3weeks) during the first 1-3 months, and less frequently (about once in 3-6 months) after that, once the child is found to be tolerating the medicine well.

Lithium carbonate has been used in children for more than two decades now, and most children tolerate it well. Potential for nephrotoxicity is the main reason that discourages clinicians and parents from the use of lithium therapy for children, though it is generally a safe drug, if the therapeutic serum level is strictly adhered to and kidney function is monitored regularly by blood tests. Lithium also has a tendency to suppress thyroid function in some youngsters, and hence, thyroid hormone levels should be monitored periodically. In areas where goiter due to iodine deficiency is endemic, lithium tends to induce goiter in some youngsters, though it is not a significant problem in the U.S. Lithium therapy is best initiated at 150 mg. twice a day in younger children and 300 mg. twice a day in the adolescent age group. Eventually it may have to be given three times a day, unless a long acting preparation that is effective at twice a day dosing is used, because of the rapid excretion of lithium. The dose is adjusted upward slowly, depending on the blood level and how well it is tolerated. The therapeutic serum level of lithium is 0.6 to 1.2 M.mol/L. The usual side effects of Lithium Carbonate are nausea, vomiting, diarrhea, and a fine hand tremor. Taking lithium after food intake can minimize the gastrointestinal side effects. Most children and adolescents attain an adequate serum level of this drug on a total daily dose of 600-1200 mg. It is best to keep the serum lithium level between 0.6–0.9 mol/L during maintenance, to minimize the possibility of acute and long-term toxicity of the drug. Dehydration will cause the serum level of the drug to rise quickly and reach toxic levels. Because of it adequate fluid intake is important for all youngsters who are given lithium. It is especially important to remember this fact during summer, because of the increased sweating and tendency for dehydration, which occur during this season.

Another medicine, not approved by F.D.A. for use in bipolar disorder, but nevertheless has been in use for many years in adults and children for treatment of the manic phase and as a maintenance treatment to prevent relapses, is the anticonvulsant, carbamazepine. Presently, it is used at times as a maintenance medicine in bipolar disorders in children, to prevent relapses in children who have failed to maintain remission with divalproex or lithium. In practice, one does not come across many children who remain fully stable for significant periods, on carbamazepine alone. The serious but rare adverse effect of carbamazepine is its tendency to produce agranulocytosis and aplastic anemia. Because of this, complete blood count before starting this medicine and periodic monitoring when the child is on this medicine are needed. Most children show a small drop in the neutrophil count when they are taking this medicine, which is considered a benign and reversible phenomenon. The serum therapeutic level of this drug is 4-12 Mcg/mL. The treatment is usually initiated with 100 to 200 mg twice a day and slowly titrated upward to reach the therapeutic level. Total doses above 900mg. per day are seldom needed to reach and maintain this therapeutic level, in children and adolescents.

Though various combinations of the mood regulators divalproex, lithium, and carbamazepine are being increasingly used in adults with intractable bipolar problems,[36] there is much less experience with such measures in children, and hence, at present, such combinations are best avoided. However, considering the fact that many children continue to be symptomatic or experience problematic relapses while taking a mood regulator with or without an additional neuroleptic, there is justification for careful use of such combinations of mood regulators, in severely ill children whose symptomatology remain at a highly problematic level. Of course, only psychiatrists who are experienced in such complex treatment modalities should undertake such measures, and that too, only with very careful monitoring.

In spite of treatment with mood regulators and neuroleptics available today, a significant percent of children suffering from bipolar disorder continue to be symptomatic or suffer from relapses, requiring further adjustments of medicines and crisis interventions, from time to time. Moreover, none of the mood regulators or neuroleptics available today prevents the occurrence of depression, which is an integral and very troublesome part of bipolar disorder.

The depressive phase of bipolar illness calls for vigilant and sensitive treatment measures. Unless delusions or hallucinations are present during the depressive phase, if the child is already on a neuroleptic because of past mania or behavioral problems, it is best to reduce or even discontinue it, because of the tendency of neuroleptics to induce or worsen depression and counteract the effects of antidepressant medicines. If a child is on maintenance mood regulators such as divalproex or lithium they are usually continued during the depressive phase. (My preference is to reduce their dose while the child is in the depressive phase.) The specific treatment for the depressive phase of bipolar disorder is treatment with antidepressant medicines. However, unfortunately, bipolar depression, often do not respond well to the antidepressants available today.

Experience with adults has shown that some people respond to one antidepressant when others do not. There is no definite method to predict who will respond to which antidepressant. Moreover, all antidepressants available today have a tendency to induce mania or hypomania in many people. All this makes the treatment of bipolar depression, often, a complex endeavor. At present, the child psychiatrist's experience in using various antidepressants in children suffering from bipolar illness and the predominant symptomatology during the depressive phase of the illness, determines the choice of antidepressant, in the treatment of bipolar depression in children.

The available methods of treating bipolar depression in children are not significantly different from the treatment of the problem in adults. The general guidelines in adults[36] are pertinent in the treatment of children also.

As in the manic, hypomanic, or related phases, the less conventional and experimental treatments are best avoided in children. Also, monoamine oxidase inhibitor (MAOI) drugs, at times used in resistant or atypical depression in adults, are best avoided in children because of the needed dietary and other precautions necessary and because of their propensity to cause serious adverse effects. Except for MAOIs, most other antidepressants available today have been in use in children during the past several years (though many are not specifically approved by F.D.A. for use in children below 12 years of age, and, as such, their use will be an off-label use). Unless the psychiatrist is very familiar with the use of a particular antidepressant in children, it is best to avoid using it without proper supervisory collaboration with another psychiatrist who has more experience in using the medicine.

Start treatment with an antidepressant known to be effective in depression and which produces the least adverse effects. Presently the selective serotonin reuptake inhibitors (SSRIs) are considered to be among the safest (but not necessarily the most effective) antidepressants to use. Fluoxentine (Prozac), paroxetine (Paxil), sertraline (Zoloft) are the main SSRIs that have been in use in children. All the SSRIs are considered to be equally effective, in general, in the treatment of depression. However, they are not as effective in bipolar depression as they are in unipolar depression. One of the reasons for this disparity may be that bipolar depression may not be based on abnormalities of serotonergic mechanisms alone, where as these medicines–the SSRIs-, are primarily supposed to address problems in that mechanism. It is quite likely that bipolar depression is caused by biochemical abnormalities involving nor-adrenergic and other not fully known mechanisms. Nevertheless, given today's limited knowledge of the biochemistry of bipolar depression and the mode of action of the antidepressants, it is wise to start treatment of a first episode of bipolar depression with an SSRI, in most cases.

The decision as to which SSRI to use may depend on the symptomatology of the depression—which could vary considerably-, and the preference of the psychiatrist as to which one may best address the symptomatology. Bipolar depression may present as an anergic depression, in which, children experience they have very little energy, motivation, or desire to engage in activities. There is also a tendency to stay in bed or home bound and sleep excessively. At times it may present as an anxious depression—one in which the sufferer feels anxious, excessively worried, or fearful about one thing or another and often, unable to rest or sleep well. In both of these general types of presentations, delusions or hallucinations may also appear.

My preference is to prescribe fluoxetine for the anergic depression and paroxetine in the anxious variety. Fluoxetine, having little sedative effect, is less likely to worsen the lethargy and hypersomnia of anergic depression. Paroxetine, on the other hand, having some sedating and anxiolytic properties, often addresses the anxiety symptoms and insomnia of anxious depression more effectively (even before the full antidepressant effect appears, which generally takes two to four weeks with almost all antidepressants). Fluoxetine is best given in the morning (if given in the evening it may produce insomnia in some children), and paroxetine is best given at night to make use of its sleep inducing properties and to avoid undue sedation during day time, especially, as most of these children are expected to be alert and function in school successfully! Sertraline is the other SSRI that has often been used in children. However, there is more uncertainty in selecting the appropriate dose of sertraline in children, compared to the other two. Fluoxetine and paroxetine are given in dosages ranging from 10—to 20 mg per day—starting at 5 to 10 mg. per day and increasing the dose gradually in one to two weeks. In my experience there is not much reason to increase the dose of these medicines above 20 mg. per day, as few children who fail to improve with four weeks of treatment with a 20mg. dose, are likely to respond to a higher dose and higher doses are more likely to produce adverse effects.

There are many children whose depression fails to respond adequately to SSRIs. The treatment of these children can be quite challenging. To chart out a course of treatment for such resistant depression the psychiatrist has to have great deal of experience in such measures. Once a child has been taking an SSRI for four weeks without appreciable improvement, whether it is better to discontinue the present antidepressant and start an antidepressant of another group, or whether adding a small dose of an antidepressant of another group to the present medicine is a better choice, is a question for which there is no clear answer. Since depression, especially bipolar depression may involve abnormalities in multiple biochemical systems—especially in the nor-adrenergic system-, it is appropriate and wise to consider an antidepressant which is considered to produce significant anti-depressant effect through its actions on more than one system. My own preference is to add very small doses of a primarily nor-adrenergic antidepressant such as desipramine (a tricyclic) to the SSRI the child is already taking, so that whatever benefit the SSRI is providing or will provide, will continue, and whatever deficiency due to its lack of action on the nor-adrenergic system would be addressed by the tricyclic. The starting dose of desipramine for such add on therapy is the smallest possible dose—10 mg. per day. Prior to starting desipramine (or any tricyclic antidepressant) in children, it is essential to obtain baseline EKG in all children and to make sure that there are no cardiac conduction problems that contraindicate their use, as tricyclic antidepressants are known to produce or worsen cardiac conduction problems—especially in children. If there is any doubt about the cardiac or EKG status of the child, obtain the opinion of a pediatric cardiologist who is familiar with the cardiac effects of tricyclics in children. In practice, most children tolerate the combination of an average dose of an SSRI and a small dose of desipramine quite well (though such combination treatment should be undertaken, only by child psychiatrists who are experienced in such treatment measures). The dose of desipramine for such add-on therapy should not exceed 25 mg. per day in younger children and 50 mg. per day in adolescents. SSRIs such as fluoxetine and paroxetine inhibit the metabolism of tricyclics through cytochrome P450 inhibition and may raise the levels of tricyclics such as desipramine 3-4 fold, and hence, special attention should be paid to possible adverse effects of tricyclics even when using such small, add-on doses. The serum level of the tricyclic should be monitored if at all possible. If the serum level is difficult to monitor because of any reason, the add-on dose of tricyclic should not exceed the 25-50 mg per day range mentioned above, and the combination therapy should not be continued if any significant adverse effect emerges. If the 25-50 mg. maximum dose of desipramine is required, it is best attained by slow weekly increments, starting with an initial dose of 10mg. per day. Many children will show an appreciable improvement within a few weeks of initiating such combination therapy. Before starting such a combination, it is essential to inform the parents (and the youngsters in an appropriate manner), that the treatment, though not contraindicated, is somewhat unconventional and why the psychiatrist is recommending such a measure. Most parents agree with such treatment measures once their concerns are addressed effectively.

As an alternative, when the child's depression appears to be resistant to an SSRI, it can be substituted with a tricyclic (after usual precautionary measures) or a non-SSRI non-tricyclic antidepressant presently available. The non-SSRI non-tricyclic antidepressants presently in use in children (off label use) are bupropion and mirtazapine. Keep in mind though that, there is only limited amount of experience with the use of these antidepressants in children at present, and hence, they should be reserved for situations where the antidepressants that have been in use longer, have proven to be ineffective.

If the SSRI has to be withdrawn and substituted with another non-MAOI antidepressant, depending on the SSRI the child is taking, the following schedule may be appropriate. Fluoxetine can be withdrawn quickly (in a few days to a week) by tapering the dose or by taking it once in two to three days only (fluoxetine discontinuation is not known to produce any withdrawal symptoms). It may not disappear from the blood fully for a week or more, however, and so there is a theoretical chance for adverse drug interactions during this period, though in general, the non-MAOI antidepressants introduced in small doses after a few days of stopping fluoxetine or when it is being withdrawn, should not produce significant problems. If the child has been taking paroxetine for quite some time, abrupt discontinuation can produce mild to moderate withdrawal symptoms, mostly in the form of nausea, vomiting, or malaise in susceptible people. Hence, it is best to taper and withdraw paroxetine gradually over a four to seven day period.

Desipramine, considering its wider therapeutic mechanisms encompassing both the noradrenergic and serotonin systems and lesser cardiovascular adverse effects compared to other tricyclics, in my experience, is the first choice among the tricyclics to treat bipolar depression. Try to keep the dose to the minimum needed to be effective, starting with a 10mg. per day dose and gradually going up to 50-75mg. if needed in pre-pubertal children and, starting at 10–20 mg. per day and going up to a maximum of 75-150mg.in adolescents. Baseline and periodic EKG monitoring is necessary in all children and adolescents who are treated with tricyclics. So also, periodic checking of serum level of the drug, especially in the initial phase of titrating the dosage, is a useful measure to provide effective dosage and avoid problematic side effects. Baseline and periodic monitoring of pulse and blood pressure is a good practice in all children treated with any tricyclic or other medicine known to produce cardiovascular side effects. It is best, to check the blood pressure both in the recumbent and standing positions to detect any problematic postural drop in blood pressure, which can cause dizziness or even fainting.

Most of the new antidepressants that have been in use in adults during the past few years have also been used in adolescents, and their success rate in this age group is generally similar to that observed in adults. Any off label use of these medicines in children and adolescents should only be undertaken with appropriate caution and only after properly informing the parents (and the youngsters also in an appropriate manner) and with their full consent. Adhering to the general principle, of starting children and adolescents on the smallest dose only of any psychotropic medicine and gradually increasing the dose with special attention paid to the possible adverse effects, is imperative.

Management of Suicidal Risk in Bipolar Depression

In my experience, the risk of suicide is higher in bipolar depression than in other types of depression. This is true with children also. Children, especially adolescents, who suffer from bipolar depression have to be carefully screened for suicide risk and appropriate precautions taken. An occasional bipolar adolescent may experience persistent and treatment resistant, severe depressive state, often accompanied by delusional thinking and hallucinatory experiences which prompt him or her to indulge in severe suicide attempts. In an occasional youngster, if pharmacological and psychotherapeutic measures fail to reverse the condition and the depression and suicidal risk remains intense, ECT may become necessary to reverse the course of the illness and save the youngster' life.

Management of Catatonia of Bipolar Depression

Another serious problem that can occur during the depressive phase of bipolar depression is the development of catatonia. **Bipolar depression has to be considered the most likely cause of catatonia in any youngster.** The tendency to consider all cases of catatonia, as a manifestation of schizophrenia only, can be treacherous in bipolar depression induced catatonia. Treatment with high doses of neuroleptics can produce disastrous consequences in such states, by worsening the catatonic phenomenon. I have personally known how such a misdiagnoses led to the death of an adolescent, who entered a hospital in a manic state misdiagnosed as schizophrenia, and who soon went into, a depressive state induced catatonia, and died due to complications of that state–the misdiagnosis having played a crucial role in the tragedy. Catatonia in bipolar depression calls for urgent measures. If treatment with antidepressants does not reverse the life threatening condition quickly, the use of ECT is fully justified.

In spite of the use of all available treatments today, many children and adults suffering from bipolar disorder will remain symptomatic and dysfunctional, to a problematic degree. The increasing use of polypharmacy (use of several medicines to treat one condition) in the treatment of bipolar disorders today, as an accepted practice, attests to this fact. Until more is known about the genetic and biochemical mechanisms underlying these disorders and specific treatment measures to correct such abnormalities become available, this sorry state of affairs is likely to continue.

The Role of Psychotherapy

Since bipolar disorder is primarily a genetic and biochemical illness, the role of psychotherapy in its treatment, is essentially, ancillary and supportive. Psychotherapy should not be considered the primary modality of treatment for bipolar disorder. This does not mean that psychotherapeutic measures are not important in the total care of the bipolar child and adult. In fact, supportive therapy by the treating psychiatrist is essential for the successful management of this illness. Because this genetic and biochemical illness primarily affects emotions, energy level, rational thinking, and even perceptions, the need for psychotherapeutic support is even more important than in other genetic, biochemical, or neurochemical illnesses, which may not primarily affect these faculties. However, **the tendency to insist that all people suffering from this disorder should take part in weekly psychotherapy sessions indefinitely, as required in many treatment settings now a days, is misguided at best and unethical at worst.**

The psychotherapeutic approach to the bipolar youngster (or adult) should be flexible, tailored to the circumstances, needs, likes, and dislikes of the individual suffering from the illness. At times there may be a greater need for, longer sessions or frequent visits with the psychiatrist or mental health professional, and at other times when the condition is more settled, the visits could and should be less frequent. Psychotherapy is mainly aimed at helping the child or adolescent live, as full and comfortable a life as possible, in a manner that is realistic, taking into consideration the nature and intensity of the illness. This includes, helping the child and family adhere to a reasonable medication regimen. Given the nature of this illness, many children—especially adolescents—and their parents, refuse to comply with treatment suggestions or drop out of treatment once the acute problems come under control. A psychotherapeutic relationship with the treating psychiatrist can help prevent such occurrences in many situations.

In toady's world, where most seriously ill bipolar children are treated in community clinic settings, often, the psychiatrist prescribes the medicines, and a psychotherapist provides psychotherapy. After an initial phase of treatment, if the symptoms have subsided significantly, many children and families find unending, weekly psychotherapy sessions unnecessary or difficult to attend regularly. The main reason for this is their often valid perception, that what transpires in the therapy sessions on an on-going basis, week after week, does not have much relevance to the symptomatology produced by the illness, which is their main concern, or certainly, they do not need such frequent sessions and visits to address whatever may be relevant to their particular situation. However, professionals often misinterpret this as "resistance" to treatment, and misunderstandings arise, with the child and parents dropping out of treatment altogether.

A flexible approach, in which, the role of psychotherapy is considered ancillary and supportive, and all treating personnel are clear in their understanding about the child's illness is essential. Such an understanding should include the awareness that, the child is in treatment for a serious mental illness caused by inherent biological abnormalities over which the child and parents have very limited control—if any. Such an approach and realistic understanding will go a long way in keeping the child and parents involved in the treatment endeavor

It will be helpful to keep in mind that the splitting of pharmacotherapy and psychotherapy between the treating psychiatrist and therapist, is mostly undertaken because of the shortage of quality psychiatric time available in the clinics where the bulk of such treatments take place. Such an arrangement is not inherently beneficial to the child or parents, and is essentially a compromise, given the less than ideal conditions that exist today in mental health treatment settings. Ideally, the treating psychiatrist should be the person conducting pharmacotherapy and psychotherapy. Others, providing case management and related services, could assist him or her. **Often, treating personnel who are not familiar with illnesses such as bipolar disorder in children, embark on a misguided approach in which they forget that the child's problems are mainly due to a biological illness that affects brain function and that the abnormal behavior and emotional turmoil are mostly a product of the illness.** Because of such misconceptions, they try to conduct psychotherapy, as if the problems are due to faulty attitudes or character defect in the child, parents, or both. The fact that many children suffering from bipolar illness exhibit conduct problems, makes the therapists forget that such conduct problems are essentially caused by the biological mechanisms that have gone awry. Many children suffering from the atypical forms of bipolar disorder behave in a self-willed and impossible to deal with manner, and even experienced professionals, including psychiatrists react to them as if they could change the way they are if only they were motivated to do so.

The approach that works best when the treatment efforts are split between a psychiatrist and psychotherapist is one, in which there is a clear understanding by both, that the child's problems are primarily due to a biological illness, and both are aware of, and agree on, the essential approach to the child's problems. The nature of interventions to be undertaken by each should be well understood and appropriate for youngsters suffering from such an illness. The teamwork and communication between the therapist and psychiatrist should be open. There should be willingness to be flexible in their approach as the situation may demand from time to time. This includes the frequency of visits to each professional to be adjusted to the needs of the child, parents, and the waxing and waning manifestations of the illness. Unfortunately, the administrative structure of many clinics, the lack of awareness by the staff as to the nature of this illness, the monetary considerations that drive the activities of the treatment settings (especially in toady's managed care environment), the power struggle between the professions, and related problems, often make such collaborations, problematic.

Keeping the best interest of the child in focus and becoming very knowledgeable about this illness, is essential, in being an effective therapist for these children. The psychiatrist and therapist should also be willing to intercede for the child and parents, with the school authorities and other agencies, when necessary, as youngsters suffering from this illness experience a great deal of school related problems, and not uncommonly, legal problems also.

Mediating between children (especially adolescents) and their parents is an often necessary and challenging task in the treatment of bipolar children. . Therapists and psychiatrists often forget that when a child (or even a parent as it often happens) is in manic, hypomanic, or a related state, he or she, is often extremely argumentative and irrationally demanding, and that it is their biological state and vulnerabilities that make them behave in such manner. Even though mediating between the child and parents is crucial when there is problematic conflict, attempting to resolve the conflict by letting–even encouraging—the child and parents have explosive arguments, in session after session, are not only unproductive but is counterproductive, and some times even down right dangerous. When a bipolar child or parent is found to be in a state of severe emotional instability, efforts should be made to bring such emotional turmoil to a more stable state or remission quickly, with the appropriate use or adjustments of medicines, while trying to maintain a reasonably peaceful atmosphere between the child and parents. **Holding, "free-for-all" type of family therapy sessions, when the bipolar participants are highly unstable emotionally and behaviorally, serves no useful purpose.** Unfortunately such out of control "family therapy" or parent-child sessions happen too often because of the lack of awareness on the part of treating personnel, as to the manifestations of bipolar disorder, and what is, and what is not appropriate for people in turmoil due to the illness. **Conflicts that cannot be resolved in the present state of emotional turmoil are best postponed for a later time when the illness is in a state of remission—when the participants will be in a state of emotional and behavioral stability and can engage in rational and appropriate interactions to resolve their conflicts.**

When the youngsters are in a state of depression, psychotherapeutic support is essential to help them continue in treatment without loosing hope and not give into self-destructive urges, if they arise. Parents need support and guidance in being supportive to the child and in not becoming overwhelmed by the child's distress and problems. Because antidepressants always take time before they become effective and combinations or several of them may have to be tried before the child recovers from the depression, parents and the child need supportive explanations often, and repeatedly, as to what is being done and what improvements could be expected, so that they will not become unduly frustrated or dejected. Mixed states of the illness pose unusual challenges in this regard as the child continues to engage in troublesome behavior while also experiencing depressive phenomena. Parents often fail to observe the depressive aspect of the youngster's symptomatology, but react harshly to the problem behavior, often making the child engage in self-destructive gestures. The therapist can help the parents become more empathic to the child's distress, by pointing out symptomatology that denote manifestations of depression or other aspects of the illness, so that the parents will not interpret the child's behavior as due to willful misbehavior. Because bipolar disorder is complex in its manifestations—especially in its atypical forms-, the treating personnel should have the expertise in identifying all its man-ifestations correctly and not mistake them for something that they are not.

The children, especially the adolescents who are insightful, often come across the understanding that the turmoil in their lives is caused by a prob-lem that is ingrained in them and over which they have little control. Often, they even note the genetic aspect of it, correctly identifying their type of symptomatology in one of the parents. Such awareness is often devastating, as it makes them face the fact that they are affected by a genetic illness that is, or can cause havoc in their lives. The therapist's capacity to understand and empathize with what the child and parents are facing, and dealing with their concerns in a supportive manner, without becoming overwhelmed is essential in such situations. Acknowledging, that the therapist understands that the illness and its troublesome mani-festations are not due to any fault of theirs and informing them of practi-cal measures that can be undertaken to alleviate the problems and predicament they are facing, may help alleviate, at least to some degree, the hopelessness which invariably accompany such situations. I find it use-ful to explain the various treatment measures that are available today, in a supportive manner, and how treatment could start with the least complex measures and how other measures could be instituted if necessary. Since parents are especially distraught that their child has become so troubled and so ill—and that too, so early in life-, and that a life of turmoil and misery await him or her, it is helpful to point out that, since the children are young, the chances of their getting the benefit of more effective reme-dies in the future are good. **I point out that there is a revolution in molec-ular biology and genetics underway and that better understanding of illnesses such as bipolar disorder and better treatment are bound to hap-pen in its sway. Encouraging the parents to join in associations and sup-port groups intended for people who suffer from bipolar disorder and their families, could be invaluable.**

The Need for Hospitalization

Out of control behavior that poses a danger to the child or others and suicidal urges that are strong are the main reasons to hospitalize a child suffering from bipolar disorder. One also takes into consideration the supportive atmosphere or lack of it at home. Some parents and families are extremely caring and reliable, but would want to avoid hospitalization. They can be counted on to help the child through the worsening phases of the illness and follow through with the recommendations of the psychiatrist fully. If there is any concern on the part of the psychiatrist that out patient treatment is insufficient because of the nature of the problem or the circumstances, it should be explained to the parents and child and, hospitalization advised. At times, it takes considerable persuasion on the part of the psychiatrist, before parents and the youngster will accept in patient hospitalization. Once hospitalization for a youngster is decided upon, further challenges await the psychiatrist and parents.

The Emergency Room Debacle

A frequent problem encountered when seeking psychiatric hospitalization for children, is the unwillingness of emergency room doctors and inpatient unit staff—especially in inner city hospitals where there is a shortage of psychiatric beds for children—to go along with the request for hospitalization. Pressures from managed care companies to avoid hospitalization, and many children not having medical insurance to cover hospitalization are other serious impediments at present. **These problems are compounded by the fact that emergency room doctors often misunderstand children, whose manic or hypomanic behavior has a conduct disorder type of presentation—the most common presentation of the atypical form of the illness-, as not being mentally ill, but only as behaving badly and being undisciplined**

In turn they develop an insensitive and rejecting attitude toward them. They look for any excuses not to admit these children to the hospital. The doctors in the emergency rooms also experience enormous pressures from other sources, not least of which is from the in-patient unit staff, who see such children as troublemakers and a bother to deal with only. Any one who has worked in such emergency rooms can recall the enormous pressures they have experienced, not to admit such children to the inpatient units. Since most bipolar children are treated in community mental health settings that are not part of hospitals with in patient facilities for children and adolescents, psychiatrists and others who work in such community clinics and treat bipolar children there, often find the whole inpatient admission process a very frustrating experience.

Sending the child to the emergency room, for in patient admission, with a well documented report pointing out why the problems of the child are due to bipolar disorder and why admission is essential, along with communicating the salient points and concerns to the emergency room staff, on the phone, will go a long way in securing the needed in patient admission for a child—even from some very impersonal settings.

As mentioned before, many children and adolescents repeatedly go through manic and hypomanic episodes in a very disruptive and dangerous manner in the community, because, admitting personnel in hospital emergency units fail to recognize the true nature of their problem. Such **doctors and others hold on to the erroneous notion that if the diagnosis they arrive upon is conduct disorder–as they often erroneously do-, the child should not be admitted to the hospital—no matter how troublesome the child's behavior.** It is not unusual to see such children send home from emergency rooms with a cursory recommendation to the parents to call the police if the child causes more trouble, or to seek out patient therapy (when the child has already been in out patient treatment and it is the treating doctor or therapist who is recommending in patient admission), or to look for a residential facility to address their "behavioral problems," when, what they urgently need is in patient hospitalization and stabilization of their turmoil due to bipolar disorder. **The plight of these children and their parents would improve tremendously, if mental** health personnel, especially those who are in charge of emergency rooms and in patient admissions become fully aware of the manifestations and ramifications of bipolar disorder–especially in its atypical form—in children and adolescents.

Understanding the problems of children who suffer from atypical bipolar disorder and to be competent in addressing their problems are perhaps the greatest skills a child psychiatrist or mental health professional working with children could possess today. My hope is that publications such as this will make at least a small contribution in accomplishing this.

AFTER WORD

I have made an attempt, to make everyone who had the desire and patience to read this book, develop at least some awareness that bipolar disorder, especially in its atypical forms, is very common in children and in my opinion, is the most urgent problem in child and adolescent psychiatry, today. I am aware that I may not have fully succeeded in accomplishing this goal. The complex nature of the problem and the present limitations in our understanding of the biology of this illness, coupled with my own limitations, I am sure, would have left many readers quite skeptical and even baffled. I hope, however, that I have succeeded, at least in raising questions in their minds, as to how frequent and serious a problem this illness may be in children. Such questioning of established thinking, I am sure, will lead each one to reach their own conclusions as they continue their helping efforts with children in one context or another.

Increased awareness, by professionals and lay people, as to how prevalent bipolar disorder is in our children, and increased understanding as to how this illness manifests in children, are essential, to bring about improvement in the plight of children affected by this illness. These children's problems and predicament affect their families, and indeed, society as a whole. Public health efforts, to make people aware of the prevalence and manifestations of this disorder, conducted in a sensitive manner, are urgently needed. Educating, mental health and other professionals who deal with children, about the prevalence and manifestations of this illness in children, and bringing about greater awareness of it, should be of the highest priority. Such awareness is sorely lacking in our universities and psychiatric centers, which train psychiatry, psychology, and social work professionals. Similar lack of awareness permeates our special educational settings and judicial venues that deal with large numbers of these children. Today's graduates from our mental health training programs, receive little exposure to the issue of bipolar disorder in children and to concepts, such as the ones articulated in this book.

It is my hope that, if members of associations such as the National Alliance for the Mentally Ill (NAMI) become more aware of the extent and seriousness of this problem, they may become advocates to promote such awareness and act as catalysts, to bring about research efforts that are urgently needed. This publication, I hope, may play a role in promoting such awareness. In coordination with the revolution in molecular biology and genetics underway presently, if intensive efforts are directed, at understanding the molecular mechanisms that cause this illness and treatment which can ameliorate them, more effective remedies–even curative and preventive ones-, may come about, in the not too distant future.

I will be more than satisfied, if this small publication will help at least a few people become truly aware of how prevalent and devastating bipolar disorder is in children and also help develop the capacity to identify children who suffer from this illness and be of service to them and their families. It would indeed be a glorious day for mankind when bipolar illness ceases to be the tragedy it is today.

REFERENCES

1. Akiskal H.S. et al., Re-evaluating the prevalence of and diagnostic composition within the broad clinical spectrum of bipolar disorders. J Affect Disord 59 (2000) S5-S30

2. American Psychiatric association. Diagnostic and Statistical Manual of Mental Disorders, Fourth Edition. Washington, DC: American Psychiatric Association; 2000

3. Avissar S et al., Differential G protein measures in mononuclear leucocytes of patients with bipolar mood disorders are state dependent. Journal Affect Disord 1997 Apr; 43(2):85-93

4. Berrettinini W.H., Pekkarinen PH., Molecular genetics of bipolar disorder. Ann. Med 28(3): 191-4, 1996 Jun

5. Blackwood D., He, L., A locus for bipolar affective disorder on chromosome 4p. Nature Genetics. Volume 12 April 1996

6. Cassano G B et al., The bipolar spectrum: a clinical reality in search of diagnostic criteria and an assessment methodology. J Affect Disord 1999 Aug 54(3): 319-28

7. Child and adolescent depression distinct from the adult version. The Brown University Child and Adolescent Behavior Letter 1995. Manisses Communications Group Inc. Providence, RI

8. Cytryn L et al., A developmental view of affective disturbances in the children of affectively ill parents. Am J Psychiatry 1984; 141:219-222

9. Davis RE., Manic-depressive variant syndrome of childhood. Am J Psychiatry 1979;136: 702-05

10. Delong G, Aldershof AL., Long-term experience with lithium treatment in childhood. J Am Acad Child Adolsc Psychiatry 1987; 26: 389-394

11. Dilsaver S C et al., Phenomenology of mania: evidence for distinct depressed, dysphoric, and euphoric presentations. Am J Psychiatry 1999 Mar; 156(3): 426-30

12. Fields A. et al., Increased cyclic AMP-dependent protein kinase activity in postmortem brain from patients with bipolar disorder. J Neurochem 1999 Oct; 73(4):1704-10

13. Freimer N., Reus V., Genetic mapping using haplotype, association and linkage methods suggests a locus for severe bipolar disorder (BPI) at 18q22-q23. Nature Genetics, Volume 12 April 1996

14. Gammon DG et al., Use of structured diagnostic interview to identify bipolar disorder in adolescent in patients. Am J Psychiatry 1983; 140:543-47

15. Ghaemi N.S., Sachs G.S. et al., Is bipolar disorder still under-diagnosed? Are antidepressants still over-utilized? Journal Affect Disord; 52(19990 135-144

16. Ginns E., Ott J. et al., A genome-wide search for chromosomal loci linked to bipolar affective disorder in the Old Order Amish. Nature Genetics; Volume 12 April 1996

17. Greenhill L.L., Pediatric Psychopharmacology, in The Clinical guide to Child Psychiatry. Scaffer, D., Ehrhardt, A.A., Greenhill, L.L. eds. The Free Press, New York, NY 1985

18. Heiden A., Association studies of candidate genes in bipolar disorders. Neuropsychobiology. Nov 2000; 42 Suppl S1: 18-21

19. Hirschfeld R M et al., Development and validation of a screening instrument for bipolar spectrum disorder: the mood disorder questionnaire. Am J Psychiatry 2000; 157 (11): 1873-5

20. Hyman SE., Goals for research on bipolar disorder: the view from NIMH. Biol psychiatry Sep 15; 48(60): 436-41

22. Isaac G., Bipolar disorder in a special educational school setting: Is it rare? J. Clinical Psychiatry 52:4, April 1991

23. Isaac G., Misdaignosed Bipolar disorder in Adolescents in a Special Educational School and Treatment Program. J.Clinical Psychiatry 53:4, April 1992

24. Isaac G., Is bipolar disorder the most common diagnostic entity in hospitalized adolescents and children. Adolescence, Vol. 30, No 118, Summer 1995

25. Kato T. et al., Association of bipolar disorder with the 5178 polymorphism in mitochondrial DNA. Am J Med Genetics 2000 Apr 3; 96(2):182-6

26. Kestenbaum CJ., Children at risk for manic-depressive illness. Am J Psychiatry 1979; 136:1206-08

27. Manji HK and Lenox RH., Signalling: cellular insights into the pathophysiology of bipolar disorder. Biol Psychiatry 2000 Sep 15; 48(6):518-30

28. Mitchell PB et al., High levels of Gs alpha in platelets of euthymic patients with bipolar affective disorder. Am j Psychiatry 1997 Feb; 154(2): 218-23

29. Neiman GW, Delong R., Use of personality inventory for children as an aid in differentiating children with mania from children with attention deficit disorder with hyperactivity. J Am Acad Child Adolesc Psychiatry 1987; 26:381-88

30. Pato C.N. et al., Genetics of bipolar disorder. CNS Spectrums 1999; 4 (6); 22-29

31. Perez J. et al., Abnormalities of cyclic adenosine monophosphate signaling in platelets from untreated patients with bipolar disorder. Arch Gen Psychiatry 1999 Mar; 56(3): 248-53

32. Post RM et al., Dysphoric mania: clinical and biological correlates. Arch Gen Psychiatry 1989; 46:353-358

33. Poznaski EO., Hypomania in a four year old. J Am Acad Child Psychiatry 1984; 23(1): 105-110

34. Risch, N., Botstein, D., A Manic-depressive History. Nature Genetics, Vol.12, April 1996

35. Rogeness GA et al., Unusual presentation of manic-depressive disorder in adolescence. J Clin psychiatry 1982; 43:37-39

36. Sachs, GS. et al., Medication treatment of bipolar disorder 2000. Postgrad Med Special Report. 2000(April): 1-104

37. Stoll AL et al., Neuroimaging in bipolar disorder: what have we learned? Biol Psychiatry 200 Sep 15; 48(6): 505-17

38. Vogt IR et al., Investigation of the human serotonin 6 receptor gene in bipolar affective disorder and schizophrenia. Am J Med Genetics 2000 Apr 3; 96(2): 217-21

39. Weller RA, Weller EB et al., Mania in pre-pubertal children. J Affect Disord 1986; 11:151-154

40. Zhan-Waxler et al., Problem behaviors and peer interactions of young children with a manic-depressive parent. Am J Psychiatry 1984; 141: 236-240

APPENDIX

(Reprinted with permission from Journal of Clinical Psychiatry, Vol. 52, no 4, April 1991)

Bipolar Disorder in Pre-pubertal Children in a Special Educational Setting: Is It Rare?
George Isaac, M.D.

The author undertook a comprehensive clinical reevaluation of five pre-pubertal children attending a special educational class for emotionally disturbed children in a day program. The children had failed to improve or had continued to worsen despite years of treatment in multiple settings. This extensive reevaluation and observation, spanning many months, revealed that all the children met DSM-III-R criteria for bipolar disorder (lifetime prevalence). None of the children had been previously diagnosed with this disorder. The author's finding suggests that bipolar disorder may be more common in severely problematic pre-pubertal children than is generally recognized. The implications of this and related issues are discussed. *(J clin Psychiatry 1991;52:165–168)*

Bipolar disorder has traditionally been considered rare in pre-pubertal children; apparently, it is rarely diagnosed or seen, even in leading psychiatric centers in the United States.[1] However, during the past few years, many clinicians have expressed their concern that bipolar disorder in children may be more common than generally perceived and that the problem may be frequently under-diagnosed or misdiagnosed.[2-7]

Clinicians with special interest in and experience with bipolar disorder have suggested that DSM-III-R criteria may have to be modified for proper identification of this problem in children.[2-4] Children diagnosed as manic have been shown to have significant family history of affective disorders.[8] A tendency for disturbance in affect regulation that appears in infancy and worsens with age, often culminating in clinically diagnosable affective illness, has been noted in studies of children of bipolar parents.[9,10] In a comparatively large sample of children studied by Akiskal et al,[5] and diagnosed bipolar by the group, none had received such a diagnosis from their previous clinicians, even though their "clinical records were replete with affective symptoms." This finding points to the possibility that the disorder is often unrecognized in children by clinicians. The atypical manner in which bipolar disorder may manifest in pre-pubertal children was noted by Davis,[6] who coined the term "manic-depressive variant syndrome of childhood." Somewhat similar observations were made the same year by Kestenbaum.[7] These authors [6,7] also emphasized the strong family history of bipolar disorder often observed in these cases and suggested that a positive family history be considered a criterion for making this diagnosis in children.

During evaluation and ongoing treatment of five pre-pubertal children who made up a class of special educational children in a day school cum treatment program, it became clear that these children had not improved in any consistent manner or were becoming worse despite years of treatment and special educational efforts in various settings. Considering this, I decided to reevaluate the children in a comprehensive manner, hoping that these reevaluations would result in a better diagnostic understanding that would lead to more appropriate treatment measures.

METHOD

I comprehensively reevaluated the five children, aged 9-11 years who made up a special education class in a day treatment program for severely emotionally disturbed children. This was undertaken because the clinical impression formed over many months was that the children remained unstable, despite present treatment and past treatment efforts in various settings. During the formal reevaluation, which spanned 4 months, I directly interviewed the children and parent(s), using a semi-structured format on multiple occasions as the clinical situation warranted.

In addition, I critically reviewed all clinical information available, recorded or otherwise, and observed the children daily in the school setting, both in and out of the classroom. During weekly formal team meetings and informal daily contacts, I obtained information from the children's therapists about their day-to-day functioning, behavior, and symptomatology. As the child psychiatrist who was present in the school setting on a full time basis, I undertook all evaluations, information gathering, and observations. These evaluation efforts were undertaken as part of the treatment efforts only and were not part of any research effort. In addition clinical information accumulated since the children entered the program was also utilized. This period of revaluation spanned a few months in the case of three children and close to two years in the case of two children.

The diagnoses resulting from the reevaluation were based on all data obtained in the present setting and additional information obtained by critically evaluating information available from previous treatment settings. The diagnosis arrived at was of "lifetime prevalence" of mental disorders, not just a diagnosis based on what was observed in the 4-month reevaluation period.

Table 1. Lifetime Prevalence of Bipolar Disorder in Five Emotionally Disturbed Prepubertal Children*

Child	Sex	Age (y)	Previous Diagnoses	Present Diagnosis	Manic Episode	Major Depressive Episode
1	M	11	Oppositional disorder, major depression	Bipolar disorder	A.C.D.E.F met; 3 of 7 met in B	Yes
2	M	11	ADHD, dysthymia, schizophrenia	Bipolar disorder mixed	A.C.D.E.F met; 4 of 7 met in B	No
3	F	11	Major depression, dysthymia	Bipolar disorder not otherwise specified	A.D.E.F met; 4 of 7 met in B	Yes
4	F	9	ADHD, atypical psychosis	Bipolar manic with psychotic features	A.C.D.E,F met; 4 of 7 met in B	Duration less than 2 wks
5	M	11	ADHD, atypical psychosis, narcissistic personality disorder, temporal lobe seizure disorder	Temporal lobe seizure disorder, bipolar disorder	A.C.D.E met; 5 of 7 met in B ? F met	NO

*Abbreviation: ADHD=attention deficit hyperactivity disorder.

** DSM-III-R criteria for manic episode (Abridged). Manic syndrome includes criteria A, B, and C. Hypomanic syndrome includes criteria A and B, but not C (marked impairment). A. Abnormally and persistently elevated, expansive or irritable mood. B. During the period of mood disturbance at least three of the following symptoms have persisted: (1) inflated self-esteem or grandiosity, (2) decreased need for sleep, (3) more talkative than usual, (4) flight of ideas, (5) distractibility, (6) increase in goal directed activity or psychomotor agitation, and (7) excessive involvement in pleasurable activities which have a high potential for painful consequences. C. Mood disturbance sufficiently severe to cause marked impairment in functioning. D. delusions or hallucinations not present as long as two weeks in the absence of prominent mood symptoms. E. Not superimposed on schizophreniform disorder, delusional disorder, or psychotic disorder not otherwise specified. F. it cannot be established that an organic factor initiated and maintained the disturbance.

FINDINGS

The findings are summarized in Table 1. The children (three boys and two girls) were aged 9-11 years. All children were of at least average intelligence, and all were living with their biological parent or parents.

Four of the five children had had psychiatric hospitalizations lasting from 2 weeks to 6 months before entering the present program. The hospitalizations were brought about in three of the children by acute worsening in their condition as manifested by agitation, over-activity, sleep changes, and dangerous impulsive behavior, which made them unmanageable at home; a fourth child (a 9-year-old girl) exhibited inappropriate excitation coupled with hyper-sexuality, auditory hallucinations, and possible delusions. The only child who did not have a history of hospitalization entered the program after her recurrent mood changes, including spells of depression and suicidal preoccupations, and other behavioral changes failed to respond to years of psychotherapeutic efforts.

The children had been involved in prior treatment efforts (mainly individual, family, and behavior therapy) for 1-5 years. At the time of entry into the program, one child was receiving methylphenidate, one an anti-depressant, and another an anti-seizure medication. None of the children had previously been diagnosed or seriously thought to be suffering from bipolar disorder. However, in the past, major depression had been diagnosed in two of the children and dysthymia in another. Three children were described as possibly "psychotic" by at least one of their clinicians during periods in which their disorder worsened. Three children had been diagnosed as having attention deficit hyperactivity disorder (ADHD). Only one child received an axis II diagnosis of developmental writing disorder. (All children had full psychological testing.) One child had a significant Axis III diagnosis of temporal lobe epilepsy.

Family history data and interviews with parents revealed that four of the five children had at least one parent who was either diagnosed as having or qualified for a diagnosis of bipolar disorder or cyclothymia. The only child for whom the diagnostic understanding of the parents was less than conclusive had grandparents with history of depression, psychotic episodes with explosive behavior, hospitalizations, and electro convulsive therapy. Thus, all five children came from families with predisposition to major mental illnesses, very likely bipolar disorder.

The reevaluation revealed that bipolar disorder was the most likely diagnosis in all five children. Since one child also suffered from temporal lobe seizure disorder, there may be some question whether this child's bipolar symptomatology could be a manifestation of his seizure disorder. Anti-seizure medications have had little impact on this child's recurrent manic and hypomanic symptoms. His father had shown evidence of hypomania on many occasions. How well the children met the DSM-III-R criteria for lifetime prevalence of bipolar disorder is summarized in Table 1.

In patients with "classical" bipolar disorder, one may expect periods of elated mania, followed by a period of full remission and discrete episodes of major depression. In general, however, these children showed a mixed and uneven pattern in which their mood periodically worsened, and they exhibited signs of dysphoric mania or mixed bipolar symptomatology; often remissions were incomplete when behavioral problems predominated. I observed at least one episode of worsening mood that could be diagnosed as mania or hypomania in each of these children. These episodic worsening of mood lasted from a few days to several weeks. The children's behavior and symptomatology during these periods differed, and there was no suggestion of "emotional contagion."

Even though the reevaluation pointed to bipolar disorder as the proper diagnosis for these children, specific treatment efforts aimed at this problem have not been easy to institute. One child was hospitalized as his dysphoric manic symptoms made him unmanageable. His symptoms appeared in the spring-time, coinciding with the timing of his hospitalization for similar problems in the preceding year. His mother agreed to a trial of lithium treatment for him based on the present findings, and this information was relayed to his treating psychiatrist in the inpatient setting.

In the other children, specific psychopharmacologic treatment aimed at bipolar disorder had not been implemented at the time of this writing for a number of reasons. I left the facility not long after making the present observations and did not have sufficient time to fully explain the new diagnostic understanding to the parents, other treatment team members, primary therapists, children's pediatricians, neurologists, and other clinicians. Most parents and others involved had been working on the assumption for years that the children's problems were due to environmental causes, ADHD, or related disorders. They expected continued psychotherapy, family therapy, behavioral measures, treatment with stimulants, or related efforts would somehow improve the condition of the children.

A history of alleged abuse by their disturbed fathers had been the ongoing focus of treatment efforts for two of the children. One child's mother was so involved in the legal issues of the alleged abuse of the child by her ex-husband that she was not ready for any other explanations for the child's disorder. The other child, who had good remissions between her brief manic episodes, had been receiving methylphenidate at the time of entry into the program, but this was discontinued when the true nature of her problem became clear. She was treated with small doses of haloperidol for a brief period when her manic symptoms intermixed with hallucinations and delusions reappeared, and the episode abated. The child's mother clearly appeared frightened and uncomfortable about long-term medications like lithium and their implications. The child's father reportedly had been prescribed lithium before the parents' traumatic separation; the mother was currently receiving antidepressant medication. Another child's mother had warned everyone concerned that her son's problems were due to his seizure disorder only and that she would not tolerate any consideration of any other diagnostic possibilities or medication.

DISCUSSION

Even though all the children met sufficient criteria to qualify for a diagnosis of bipolar disorder, clearly, in pre-pubertal children, the symptom criteria have to be examined and interpreted, taking into consideration the child's developmental level. Unlike adults who are manic, children of this age group are unlikely to engage in buying sprees, foolish business investments, or other examples of manic behavior given in DSM-III-R.

Some behavior patterns exhibited by these children do resemble the behavior patterns of children with conduct and impulse control problems in general. However, the severe intensity of the problems and their periodic acute worsening to crisis proportions when these children appear to lose all control, as well as accompanying agitation and changes in sleep patterns, appetite, and energy level point to bipolar disorder as the correct diagnosis. These children, more often than not, exhibited mixed or dysphoric and, thus, atypical forms of mania or hypomania during acute periods of worsening, which may account for some of the past misdiagnosis of this problem. The finding is in keeping with the observations of Akiskal et. Al.[5] Adults when manic often act like excited or very angry children. Similar phenomena appearing in children may require much more careful observation and evaluation over longer periods of time and throughout multiple episodes before the true nature of the problems become clear. In the present group of children, no other DSM-III-R diagnosis could have explained the intense, recurring, and varied psychopathology these children exhibited over many years.

The finding that five of five pre-pubertal children met criteria for bipolar disorder on careful scrutiny points to the possibility that bipolar disorder may be much more common in such children than has been recognized. Measures that may be helpful in the proper diagnosis of such children include (1) a careful review of history and lifetime symptomatology and behavior patterns; (2) prolonged periods of careful observation; (3) careful documentation of family history of psychiatric disorders, especially bipolar disorder, preferably by direct interview and observations; (4) awareness of the occurrence of bipolar disorder in this age group, especially in its atypical, dysphoric, and mixed forms, as well as awareness of incomplete remissions; (5) careful reevaluation of children previously diagnosed with ADHD, who begin to show spells of depressive episodes and episodes of acute behavioral worsening and show no consistent improvement with stimulants and other usual treatment measures for ADHD.

Since the present diagnosis of bipolar disorder was arrived at mainly by the efforts of one evaluator only, inadvertent bias toward over-diagnosis of the problem cannot be ruled out. My findings may not be representative of the problems of young children in similar settings. The present group of children were specially referred to and accepted into the program because they were understood to be severely dysfunctional children who had failed to improve with efforts in other special educational settings. Nevertheless, the finding that bipolar disorder was seldom if ever considered a possibility in these children during their many years of unsuccessful treatment, including hospitalizations, appears to be significant. It is likely that the previous clinicians did not have the opportunity to do as intense and prolonged a study as was possible in the present setting.

The diagnosis of bipolar disorder presents, the child psychiatrist, and other clinicians with many complex dilemmas, as was evident from my preliminary experience with the parents of this group of children. These and elated factors interfere with proper treatment. Parents often resist and are frightened of such a diagnosis; this reaction is compounded by the fact that, for years, treatment efforts have proceeded with the understanding that the children's problems were caused by environmental factors or were manifestations of ADHD only. The concept of bipolar disorder in young children is new to many, mental health and medical professionals, and there may be resistance to accepting this idea. The fact that many parents themselves may suffer from this disorder, as seen in this study, adds immensely to the complexity of the problem. The parents are often volatile, and their capacity to deal with this type of problem in their children appears limited.

These preliminary and limited findings emphasize the need for the mental health and medical community to become more aware of these issues, so that more well thought out studies are instituted and strategies to help these children and their families are developed.

Drug names: haloperidol (Haldol and others), methylphenidate (Ritalin).

REFERENCES

1. Greenhill LL. Pediatric psychopharmacology. In: Schaffer D, Ehrhardt AA, Greenhill LL, Eds. The Clinical Guide to Child Psychiatry New York, NY: The Free Press; 1985

2. DeLong RG, Aldershof AL. Long-term experience with lithium treatment in childhood. J Am Acad Child Adolesc psychiatry 1987; 26(3): 389-394

3. Poznanski EO, Israel MC, Grossman J. hypomania in a four year old. J Am acad child psychiatry 1984; 23(1): 105-110

4. Weller RA, Weller EB, Tucker SG, et al. Mania in pre-pubertal children. J Affective Disord 1986; 11: 151-154

5. Akiskal HS, Downs J, Jordan P, et al. Affective disorders in referred children and younger siblings of manic-depressives. Arch Gen Psychiatry 1985; 42: 996-1003

6. Davis RE. Manic-depressive variant syndrome of childhood. Am J Psychiatry 1979; 136: 702-706

7. Kestenbaum CJ. Children at risk for manic-depressive illness. Am J Psychiatry 1979; 136: 702-706

8. Neiman GW, De Long R. Use of personality inventory for children as an aid in differentiating children with mania from children with attention deficit disorder with hyperactivity. J Am Acad Child Adolesc Psychiatry. 1987; 26(3): 381-388

9. Zahn-Waxler C, M$_c$ Knew DH, Cummings EM, et al. Problem behaviors and peer interactions of young children with a manic-depressive parent. Am J Psychiatry 1984; 141: 236-240

10. Cytryn L, McKnew DH, Zahn-Waxler C, et al. A developmental view of affective disturbances in the children of affectively ill parents. Am J Psychiatry 1984; 141: 219-222

Reprinted with permission from The Journal of Clinical Psychiatry, vol. 53,no. 4, April 1992

Misdiagnosed Bipolar Disorder in Adolescents in a Special Educational School and Treatment Program

George Isaac, M.D.

Background: twelve adolescents found to be the most problematic, crisis prone, and treatment resistant were comprehensively revaluated in the special educational day school and treatment program they were attending. This evaluation took place over a 6-month period and was done to arrive upon a comprehensive diagnostic understanding so that more relevant and effective treatment measures could be instituted.

Method: The author conducted semi-structured interviews with the adolescents on multiple occasions as the clinical situation warranted. All information available, recorder or otherwise, was comprehensively reviewed and reevaluated. The children were observed informally in and out of their classrooms throughout the period. All parents available were interviewed to clarify the children's present and past symptomatology and to assess the nature of psychiatric disorders, if any, in first—and second-degree family members.

Results: the reevaluation showed that 8 of the 12 youngsters clearly satisfied DSM-III-R criteria for bipolar disorder, which had been misdiagnosed mainly as attention-deficit hyperactivity disorder (ADHD) and conduct disorder. Three other youngsters showed significant bipolar features though not fully satisfying the criteria for this disorder.

Conclusions: Bipolar disorder may be very common among highly problematic adolescents in special educational and outpatient treatment facilities for emotionally disturbed youngsters but may still be misdiagnosed very often as ADHD and conduct disorder, with all the negative consequences of such misdiagnosis.

(Journal of Clinical Psychiatry 1992; 53: 133-136)

While attempting to offer effective psychiatric treatment for adolescents enrolled in a therapeutic special educational day school for emotionally disturbed students, the staff noted that the functioning of some of the youngsters had improved little or was even worsening despite prolonged treatment and special educational efforts in various settings in the past. Some of the youngsters were proving difficult to manage in the school, home, or community and were highly crisis prone. As the full-time child psychiatrist, I comprehensively reevaluated the most problematic of the youngsters in the school setting over a 6-month period. This paper is based on the findings that emerged as a result of the reevaluation.

During the past two decades it has been repeatedly pointed out that bipolar disorder is often under-diagnosed or mistaken for other disorders in adolescents, such as attention-deficit hyperactivity disorder (ADHD), conduct disorder, or adolescent turmoil.[1-7] Most of these reports have come from inpatient, academic, or research centers; as far as I know, this problem has not been identified in groups of children in community special educational settings.

A study[8] of large group of children with varied diagnoses who were being treated with lithium suggested that some of their behavioral problems like aggressiveness, explosiveness, and mood lability might have been related to bipolar disorder. The importance of family history of diagnosed and undiagnosed bipolar disorder in the proper recognition of this disorder in children has been pointed out by others.[2,5-8] The fact that bipolar disorders often produces problematic personality dysfunctioning due to incomplete remissions[9] and that mania often presents with dysphoric features rather than elation and euphoria[10] was pointed out in studies on adults recently. That bipolar disorder frequently presents in adolescents as a chronic illness with mixed features and not just as an episodic illness has been highlighted by Akiskal and Weller.[11]

METHOD

Of approximately 50 children enrolled in a special educational school for emotionally disturbed children, 12 adolescents were comprehensively reevaluated. Children who attended this school had a history of being unmanageable because of their emotional and behavioral problems in less intensive therapeutic school settings. All children were classified as emotionally disturbed for educational purposes. The 12 children were selected for reevaluation as they were found to require frequent crisis interventions, in a majority of cases because of their severely disruptive behavior. They appeared to be at high risk for having to be removed from or dropping out of the program. They were in general unresponsive to the psychotherapeutic, behavioral, and pharmacological measures that had been implemented in the present setting and elsewhere. The reevaluations were undertaken for clinical purposes only and were not part of any research efforts.

Over a 6-month period, I interviewed all children using a semi-structured format on multiple occasions as the clinical situation warranted. In addition, I interviewed the children's parents or parent at least once and in most cases on more than one occasion to clarify the youngsters' past and present symptomatology and response to treatment measures; to assess the mental functioning of the parent; and to assess the nature of psychopathology, if any, in other first and second degree relatives, using the family history method. I gathered information from the children's therapists and teachers formally during weekly team meetings and informally on other days when needed and observed the children in and out of the classroom informally and an ongoing basis. All past information available, recorded or otherwise, was critically reviewed. Based on all these efforts, I arrived at a lifetime diagnosis of mental disorders using DSM-III-R[12] criteria.

RESULTS

The findings are summarized in table 1. The youngsters (10 males, 2 females) were from 13 to 19 years of age and were of at least average intelligence. Eleven were white and one was Hispanic. The reevaluation revealed two major diagnostic groups: bipolar disorder (N=8) and conduct disorder, possibly bipolar related (N=3). One child was diagnosed as possibly having schizoaffective disorder.

Bipolar Disorder

Eight youngsters qualified for a definite lifetime diagnosis of DSM-III-R bipolar disorder. Four showed discrete periods of manic or hypomanic episodes interspersed with short-lived or mild depressive episodes and reasonably good remissions in between; 3 showed dysphoric or mixed bipolar symptomatology, often with rapid cycling and incomplete remissions, making their management difficult most of the time and extremely difficult during the acute worsening, and 1 was prone to recurrent episodes of severe depression with psychotic features between the brief manic episodes.

Table 1. Summary of Findings in 12 Treatment Resistant Adolescents in a Special Educational Day School

No	Sex	Age	Previous Diagnoses	Present Diagnosis	Suicidal Tendency	Family History	History of Stimulant Treatment
1	M	19	Conduct disorder, Organic personality disorder	Bipolar disorder	Attempt (hanging)	Alcoholism	No
2	M	19	ADHD, Borderline, Drug-induced psychosis	Bipolar disorder	Rumination	Bipolar	No
3	F	17	Major depression with psychosis	Bipolar disorder	Gesture/preoccupation	Psychosis/bipolar	No
4	M	15	ADHD, schizophrenia, schizoaffective	Bipolar disorder	Threats	Depression, panic disorder, ? bipolar	Yes
5	M	18	Conduct disorder, dysthymic disorder	Bipolar disorder	…	Cyclothymia, ? bipolar	NO
6	M	18	Conduct disorder	Bipolar disorder	Attempt (hanging)	Bipolar	No
7	M	16	ADHD. Conduct disorder, depression	Bipolar disorder	Threats	Depression/ agoraphobia, ? bipolar	Yes
8	M	16	Conduct disorder, ?drug induced psychosis	Bipolar disorder	…	Bipolar Nos	No
9	F	14	Schizophrenia, depression	?Schizoaffective disorder	Gestures	Psychosis, ? bipolar	No
10	M	13	ADHD, conduct disorder, depression	Conduct disorder (? Bipolar related)	Threats	Alcoholism, Violence ? bipolar	Yes
11	M	14	ADHD, conduct disorder, depression	Conduct disorder (?bipolar related)	Threats	Not available (adopted)	Yes
12	M	15	ADHD, conduct disorder	Conduct disorder (?bipolar related)	Preoccupations, threats	Cyclothymia, depression, alcoholism	Yes

*Abbreviations: ADHD=attention-deficit hyperactivity disorder, NOS=not otherwise specified

In 7 of 8 bipolar youngsters, I observed at least one episode of mania or hypomania while they were in the present program. Four exhibited grandiose delusions when manic. Episodes of major depression satisfying

DSM-III-R criteria seemed to have occurred in only one of the 8. However, 7 of these 8 youngsters reported suicidal ruminations from time to time. Two of the 7 had attempted suicide by hanging in the past and 2 others had made less serious attempts.

Episodes of dysphoria or depression lasting a few days were often noted in some youngsters. Their functioning during these brief periods was markedly different from their usually boisterous, defiant, high-energy existence. They complained of feeling "dizzy," "dumb," "weird," and "stupid," being in a "fog" and not being able to "think" during these episodes and often sought out members of the staff for comfort. Six of the youngsters have had criminal charges against them. Four were known to abuse alcohol or marijuana at times.

Conduct Disorder possibly Related to Emerging Bipolar Disorder

Three children, aged 13-15 years, were diagnosed as having conduct disorder that was possibly an initial manifestation of an emerging bipolar disorder. As in the majority of the youngsters in the bipolar group, externalizing behavior problems, episodes of behavioral worsening, emotional lability, and suicidal threats or ruminations were common in these youngsters also. Generally, the conduct problems were more or less continuous in these youngsters and periodically worsened. However, the features suggestive of mania or depression in these children were not extensive enough to satisfy DSM-III-R criteria for bipolar disorder, and the severe conduct problems, impaired functioning, and nature and quality of mood changes could not fit a diagnosis of cyclothymia.[12] Hence the diagnosis of these three children continued to be conduct disorder with the strong possibility that they were manifesting early signs of a bipolar disorder.

Family History

Of the 11 youngsters in the bipolar and conduct disorder, possibly bipolar related, groups, 9 had a first-and/or second-degree relative who either definitely or very likely suffered from bipolar disorder or a major mental disorder with strong affective components. Seven of the 9 had a parent who was noted to be or reported to be suffering from symptomatology highly suggestive, if not conclusive, of bipolar disorder or cyclothymia.

Previous Diagnoses and Treatment Measures

All 12 youngsters had received treatment in various mental health facilities for the last 1 to 10 years. Ten had one or more psychiatric hospitalizations in the past. Seven out of the 8 bipolar disorder youngsters had received the diagnosis of ADHD and conduct disorder repeatedly in the past, and most of their treatment had been dictated by such diagnoses. It was evident from their past history and records that they continued to receive such diagnoses even after their bipolar symptomatology had manifested clearly. Bipolar disorder was mentioned as a differential diagnostic possibility in only 2 of these 7 youngsters in the past, but little attempt was made to explore this possibility further. Three youngsters who had experienced hallucinations or delusions in the past received the diagnosis of schizophrenia, borderline personality, and drug induced psychosis (not supported by laboratory data or history from the patient), respectively, and their bipolar symptoms seemed to have gone unrecognized during these periods.

Five of the 7 youngsters had been treated with stimulants in the past for periods varying from many months to several years, for their presumed ADHD problems. Although, treatment with stimulants was often restarted by clinicians who saw the youngsters in crisis situations, there was little evidence that the stimulants were of benefit.

All 12 youngsters had received various forms of psychotherapeutic (individual, group, family) and behavioral treatment for varying periods from various facilities in the past. Nine had been enrolled in various special educational programs, and 3 of the 12 had even lived in residential treatment centers.

Four of the 12 youngsters had previously received small-to-moderate doses of neuroleptics, but none remained stable for long periods on neuroleptic treatment alone as their symptomatology changed, waxed and waned.

DISCUSSION

That 8 of 12 highly problematic adolescents qualified for a definite diagnosis of bipolar disorder as a result of this reevaluation is an important finding that may have significant relevance to the understanding and treatment of such youngsters in similar and related settings. No other DSM-III-R diagnosis could have sufficiently explained the varied waxing and waning, internalizing and externalizing symptomatology these youngsters exhibited, often through many years.

The finding strongly suggests that bipolar disorder is *quite common* among problematic adolescents but is *still* being misdiagnosed often as conduct disorder, ADHD, or other disorders, with all the negative consequences of such misdiagnosis. As a result of misdiagnosis, the youngsters are denied trials of possibly effective treatment measures, are often seen as willfully "bad," and may be subjected to treatment measures that are not only ineffective but also possibly harmful, like continued treatment with stimulants.

It is possible that the previous clinicians who dealt with these youngsters did not have the opportunity to observe them for as prolonged and intensive a manner as was possible during the present reevaluation, which would account for bipolar disorder not being recognized by many in the past. It is also understood that clinicians who saw these children before the disorder manifested fully could not have seriously suspected that they were observing early signs of bipolar disorder. It has to be emphasized, however, that the evidence showed that 7 of the 8 bipolar patients had been seen by clinicians in outpatient and/or inpatient settings after the illness manifested in an identifiable form, but the problem of misdiagnosing continued. This is in keeping with the observations of others.[1,3,6,7,11]

The following points, based on the present findings and opinions artic-ulated by others previously,[1,3,4,6,7,11] may be helpful in the proper recog-nition of bipolar disorder in adolescents:

1. A heightened awareness that bipolar disorder is quite common in highly problematic adolescents.

2. Bipolar disorder may manifest not just as an episodic illness exhibiting elation or depression but very often as an illness marked by incom-plete remissions, waxing and waning symptomatology, and mixed and dysphoric features that mimic a disruptive behavior disorder.

3. The proper identification of the disorder may require prolonged periods of ongoing observation by the same clinician or team along with periodic semi-structured interviews of the youngsters and primary caregivers covering the features of mania, hypomania, and depression—not only in its classical form but also in its mixed, atypical, and dysphoric forms.

4. The family history of bipolar disorder in first–and second-degree family members should be clarified and recognized, preferably by direct interviews and observations.

5. The diagnostic significance of brief depressions, periodic somatic symptoms, and low energy states in children diagnosed as having ADHD and conduct disorder, especially in those who have not responded to usual treatment measures for such problems, should be carefully evaluated.

6. All adolescents manifesting major depression or psychotic features should be observed for possible shifts into often transient manic or hypomanic behavior.

Four of the children—including one from the conduct disorder, possibly bipolar related group—were placed on a regimen of lithium as a result of this reevaluation, with moderate-to-good results (one youngster with a high I.Q. who had been repeatedly dismissed from many schools because of his periodic behavioral worsening has now graduated from high school and entered college). This does not imply that all these youngsters would be lithium responsive.

Since I left the day school not long after completing this work, there was insufficient time to impress many of the parents, youngsters, and involved clinicians with the need to change the treatment strategy in accordance with these findings. This problem is compounded by the fact that many of the parents themselves are affectively unstable and also nurture the hope–often reinforced by well-meaning clinicians–that the youngsters will grow out of their problems as they become older.

The fact that all these reevaluations and re-diagnosing were undertaken by one child psychiatrist (author) only raises the possibility that an inadvertent tendency on the part of this clinician to over-diagnose bipolar disorder cannot be ruled out. Nevertheless the finding of a very high prevalence of bipolar disorder in this selected group of adolescents that went undetected until now points to the need for mental health clinicians, especially psychiatrists and child psychiatrists, to become more aware of the nature and manifestations of bipolar disorder in adolescents.

REFERENCES

1. Gammon DG, John K, Rothblum DE, et al. Use of structured diagnostic interview to identify bipolar disorder in adolescent inpatients. Am J psychiatry 1983: 140: 543-547

2. Rogness GA, Reister AE, Wicoff JS. Unusual presentation of manic-depressive disorder in adolescence. J Clin psychiatry 1982; 43: 37-39

3. Neiman GW, Delong R. Use of the personality inventory for children as an aid in differentiating children with mania from children with attention deficit disorder with hyperactivity. J Am acad Child adolesc psychiatry 1987; 26: 381-388

4. Carlson GA, Strober M. Affective disorder in adolescence: issues in misdiagnosis. J Clin Psychiatry 1978; 39: 59-66

5. Kestenbaum CJ. Children at risk for manic-depressive illness. Am J Psychiatry 1979; 136: 1206-1208

6. Davis RE. Manic-depressive variant syndrome of childhood. Am J psychiatry 1979; 136: 702-705

7. Akiskal HS, Downs J, Jordan P, et al. Affective disorders in referred children and younger siblings of manic-depressives. Arch Gen Psychiatry 1985; 42: 996-1003

8. Delong G, Aldershof AL. Long term experience with lithium treatment in childhood. J Am Acad Child Adolesc psychiatry 1987; 26: 389-394

9. Harrow M, Goldberg JF, Grossman LS, et al. Outcome in manic disorders. Arch Gen Psychiatry 1990; 47: 665-671

10. Post RM, Rubinow DR, Uhde TW, et al. Dysphoric mania: clinical and biological correlates. Arch Gen psychiatry 1989; 46: 353-358

11. Akiskal HS, Weller EB. Mood disorders and suicide in children and adolescents. In: Kaplan HI, Sadock BJ eds. Comprehensive Text Book of psychiatry. 5th ed. Baltimore, Md: Williams & Wilkins; 1989: 1981-1994

12. American Psychiatric Association. Diagnostic and statistical manual of Mental disorders, Third edition, Revised. Washington, DC: American psychiatric association; 1987

Previously published in Adolescence, Vol. 30, No. 118, summer 1995

IS BIPOLAR DISORDER THE MOST COMMON DIAGNOSTIC ENTITY IN HOSPITALIZED ADOLESCENTS AND CHILDREN

George Isaac

An evaluation of all children and adolescents admitted to an acute psychiatric unit over a three-month period was undertaken to determine the presence of bipolar disorder. The findings indicated that bipolar disorder was the most common diagnostic entity. This disorder had not been recognized in most of these youngsters previously, although almost all of them have had past psychiatric contacts. The vast majority of youngsters experiencing delusions and / or hallucinations, and the vast majority of court-remanded adolescents also appeared to be suffering from this disorder. It was concluded that bipolar disorder has to be ruled out in all youngsters admitted to acute care psychiatric units.

INTRODUCTION

Several studies have brought attention to the fact that bipolar disorder is often unrecognized or misdiagnosed in children and adolescents as attention deficit hyperactivity disorder (A.D.H.D.), conduct disorder, adolescent turmoil, and other disorders (Akiskal et al., 1985; Akiskal & Weller, 1989; Carlson, 1990; Davis, 1979; Delong & Aldershof, 1987; Gammon, John, & Rothblum, 1983; Isaac, 19991; Isaac, 1992; Neiman 7 Delong, 1987). In two previous studies conducted by the author (Isaac, 1991, 1992) it was observed that bipolar disorder is very common but often unrecognized in the most problematic children and adolescents in a day school and treatment program for severely emotionally disturbed youngsters. As a result, a comprehensive evaluation of all children and adolescents admitted to a 14-bed child and adolescent psychiatry unit of a county general hospital in New York state was undertaken to determine the presence of this disorder. This paper reports the findings of that evaluation.

METHOD

All children and adolescents admitted to the unit during a three-month period (March-May 1992 were evaluated with special attention paid to the possibility that bipolar disorder would be the primary diagnosis in some or many of these patients. Measures found to be useful in identifying this disorder in this age group as summarized in the author's previous papers on the subject (Isaac. 1991, 1992) and pointed out by others (Akiskal; et al., 1985; Akiskal & Weller 1989; Carlson 1990; Davis, 1979; Delong & Aldershof, 1987) were applied. These included repeated semi-structured interviews by the author, as clinically warranted, to elicit present or past experiences and symptoms which would be indicative of bipolar disorder, careful observation of the patients throughout their hospital stay, gathering information from other staff members, obtaining a history of patients' lifetime symptomatology with special attention to episodes suggestive of mania, hypomania, and depression, especially in those previously diagnosed as suffering from A.D.H.D. and conduct disorder. In addition, gathering of family history data either by interviewing immediate family members or eliciting data on family history suggestive of the disorder through a reliable close relative was also undertaken. These efforts were part of a comprehensive clinical evaluation and not performed primarily for research purposes.

FINDINGS

Fifty-seven patients (age-range 7-17 years; 32 males, 25 females; 29 white, 24 black, 4 others) were admitted during this period. Of these patients, 13 were pre-pubertal (below 13 years of age). Seventeen admissions had been court remanded for psychiatric evaluations. All except one of these youngsters were post-pubertal.

Fourteen youngsters (including five pre-pubertal children) met the DSM III R criteria for bipolar disorder fully (referred to hereafter as the "definitely bipolar" group). Fifteen other children appeared to have features and a history highly suggestive of bipolar group (referred to hereafter as "very likely bipolar" group) but not meeting the DSM III R criteria fully at present. Fourteen children seemed to warrant prolonged observation and study to rule out the possibility of bipolar disorder (which was not possible at that time because of their very short stay, mostly for administrative reasons).

Thirteen of the 17 court-remanded youngsters were in the definitely or very likely bipolar groups. Eight of the ten (including five pre-pubertal) who showed psychotic phenomena (hallucinations and /or delusions) were in the definitely bipolar group.

Until the evaluation took place, most of the youngsters considered as belonging to the definitely or very likely bipolar groups had had a diagnosis of conduct disorder, attention deficit hyperactivity disorder or adjustment disorder. In very few, if any, of these youngsters, had a diagnosis of bipolar disorder been entertained as a serious possibility according to past records.

The definitely or very likely group accounted for more than 50% of the patients. This percentage did not include those youngsters who were in need of further observation in order to rule out a diagnosis of bipolar disorder. Categorizing children and adolescents as very likely bipolar, appears to be justified since in the early stages they often go through periods when the symptomatology is not fully manifest in the classical adult form. Further, no other DSM III R diagnosis can explain the past varied symptomatology and behavior of these children. During the same period, a year before this focused evaluation, only five children had been diagnosed with bipolar disorder in the same unit.

Twelve youngsters from the definitely and very likely groups were treated with medication (Lithium, Carbamazepine, and or neuroleptics) for the disorder, which produced good results in nine of them, including three who were switched from stimulants because of poor response and the new diagnostic understanding.

DISCUSSION

The findings here point to the strong possibility that (1) Bipolar disorder is not only not uncommon (Gammon, et al., 1983) but may be the *most common diagnostic entity* in children and adolescents in similar settings. (2) Most youngsters noted to be experiencing or having experienced psychotic phenomena and admitted to such settings may be suffering from bipolar disorder. (3) It may be the most common diagnosis in adolescents who are court-remanded to such settings. (4) Bipolar disorder may still be going unrecognized and misdiagnosed in a majority of youngsters who suffer from it.

The finding that the vast majority of court-remanded adolescents admitted to the unit were in definitely or very likely groups, raises the possibility that such youngsters often may be entangled in the legal system, rather than receiving the understanding and treatment they actually require.

The finding that most of the patients who experienced delusions or hallucinations belonged to the definitely bipolar group, points to the strong possibility that the disorder may be the underlying cause of such psychotic phenomena in most children and adolescents admitted to similar acute-care settings. As far as the author is aware, the possibility of such a strong connection has not been reported previously.

It should be noted that because evaluations and final diagnoses were made primarily by the author, there is the strong possibility of an inadvertent tendency to over-diagnose bipolar disorder in these youngsters. However, if these preliminary findings are supported by studies in other similar settings, they may have profound implications for understanding and treatment of children and adolescents.

REFERENCES

Akiskal, HS., Downs, J., & Jordan, P. (1985). Affective disorders in referred children and younger siblings of manic-depressives. Archives of General Psychiatry, 42, 996-1003.

Akiskal, HS., & Weller EB,. (1989) Mood disorders and suicide in children and adolescents. In H.L. Kaplan, & B.J. Sadock, (Eds.) Comprehensive Text Book of Psychiatry. 5th ed. Baltimore, Md: Williams& Wilkins.

Carlson, GA (1990). Bipolar disorder in children and adolescents. In B.D. Garfenkel, G.A. Carlson, & E.B. Weller (eds.). Psychiatric disorders in children and adolescents. Philadelphia: W.B. Saunders.

Davis, R.E. (1979). Manic-depressive variant syndrome of childhood. American journal of Psychiatry, 136, 1206-1208.

Delong, G., & Aldershof, A.L. (1987). Long term experience with lithium treatment in childhood. Journal of American Academy of Child & Adolescent Psychiatry., 26, 389-394.

Gammon, D.G., John, K., Rothblum, D.E. (1983). Use of structured diagnostic interview to identify bipolar disorder in adolescent inpatients. American Journal of Psychiatry, 140, 543-547.

Isaac, G., (1991). Bipolar disorder in pre-pubertal children in a special educational setting: Is it rare? Journal of Clinical Psychiatry, 52, 165-168.

Isaac, G., (1992) Misdiagnosed bipolar disorder in adolescents in a special educational school and treatment program. Journal of Clinical Psychiatry, 53, 133-136.

Neiman, G.W.., & Delong R. (1987). Use of the personality inventory in children as an aid in differentiating children with mania from children with attention deficit disorder with hyperactivity. Journal of American Academy of Child and Adolescent Psychiatry, 26, 381-388

0-595-21091-0